THE FITTER CONFIDENT YOUNIVERSE

AN LGBTQ+ GUIDE TO WELLBEING ON OUR TERMS

MATT BOYLES

CONTENTS

DEDICATION

Dedicated to Fitter, Confident Younicorns everywhere.

A rising tide lifts all boats…

(Lots of people, including me!)

INTRODUCTION

Welcome to The Fitter Confident Youniverse: an LGBTQ+
Guide to Wellbeing on Our Terms

Ahoy! Thank you SO much for buying this book; that means
another £1 is going to the Albert Kennedy Trust, a really
wonderful charity that supports vulnerable young LGBTQ+
people, getting them off the streets, in education and training
and giving them a far brighter future.

If you *didn't* buy it and have borrowed this copy, well why not
consider donating £1 their way, to keep the goodness this
book is doing, flowing? (more on AKT at the back.)

This book - my sort-of first - will take you on a journey to help
you know how to build a Fitter, Confident You... *on your terms.*
This is what I've been doing for more than 11 years, and I'm
ridiculously proud to say I've worked with more than 1,400
clients all around the world.

But what does *'on your terms'* mean? Outlining what this book will do for you, who it's for and how it will help would be pretty useful at this stage... So, let's do that now.

I am a gay man (sorry ladies!!!) who discovered the power of having a bit of fitness and wellbeing in his life. I'm 41 now (as of August 2022, when this book was first published) and am the fittest, strongest, healthiest and most confident I've ever been.

On one hand, that might seem logical: the more time you have... Well, the more time you have to learn, grow, workout, eat better and so on.

But of course, life isn't logical. And while time is linear (as far as we know), with the best intentions in the world, there are always curveballs, both big and small, to throw us off track.

But before we even get to me and my curveballs (don't ask, sensitive area - literally), let's take a step back and look at what's going on for us all. Let's imagine a world without Covid for a second - a lovely thought, I'm sure you'll agree - as what I want to discuss pre-dates the pandemic.

Allow me to introduce a 46-year-old man named George. He's outwardly happy (enough). He has regular employment in an office job that he doesn't mind. He has a partner of 5 years and they're pretty ok together. They have a car and they own a two-bed house in Reading and go on a couple of holidays a year (when allowed). George walks to work a few times a week, but also works long hours some days, so when the weekend comes, he believes he's earned his downtime and he has a quiet few days, not doing much - might see friends, might go to the cinema or out for a meal.

At New Year he joined a gym as he noticed his trousers getting a bit tighter, and he only bought new ones in a size up last year. He gamely throws himself into it, hitting the treadmill for a soul-sapping 30 minutes and then forcing himself onto the exercise bike too, as he knows cardio is good to burn fat.

Walking onto the gym floor brings back some formative memories of his school years: feeling unfit, not being good at football (not really enjoying it either, but there were no other options in the 80s). There was also a PE teacher who made up a nickname for him he can't quite remember, but the teacher *always* used it, which was embarrassing. It wasn't an insult as such, but he always felt singled out and being picked last or almost-last did nothing for his confidence around fitness and sport.

It was also around this time that George started to feel different, in a way he couldn't pinpoint. Looking back, of course it was because he's gay, but in the pressure cooker of a 1980s all boys school, it was pushed to the back of the list of things to overthink.

George and his partner decide they both need to change their eating habits too, as they've been over-reliant on takeaways and convenience foods - what used to be reserved just for a Friday 'treat' has become multiple times a week - he's recently noticed the cost too. They cut out alcohol and anything sweet as well and push on through the withdrawal headaches they get in the first few days, which are then replaced with chew-your-hand-off hunger pains - even though George is having the healthy cereal advertised by that Olympian...

George and his partner make it through the first week... But they're miserable. They're snapping at each other; both have low moods and he's not sleeping well either. But hey! He's lost 2lb, so that's good, isn't it? And he pushes into the second week.

But work is particularly busy for George this week; he has to finish a report for this Quarter, while training a new member of his team and doing his regular work. So, the late nights kick in again, and while he had the best will in the world to exercise before work, the treadmill didn't seem as appealing as his bed when the alarm went off at 6.15 in the morning...

Plus, he's never felt very comfortable in the gym - he feels out of place, that people are watching him (so he tries to make it look like he's working really hard on the treadmill - he's certainly sweating lots, so it must be working), the PTs spoke to him at first but after he didn't buy any sessions with them, they lost interest.

The gym also forces him up close and personal with other gym-goers, all who clearly know what they're doing, and lifting what look like enormous weights. He wonders if he's the only gay man who doesn't have a six pack or workout six days a week; it certainly feels that way sometimes.

It's also sweaty and the showers don't seem to have been cleaned for at least a week (the same chewing gum and plaster were in the drain of the shower which he spotted the week before), so he hits snooze and sleeps for another 45 minutes.

He still wakes up groggy and feeling a bit sluggish, but that's what life is like in your 40s, isn't it? Most of his friends agree, so he just puts up with it and goes to work.

The work is particularly tiring and concentration-heavy and George doesn't have the energy or the time to workout this week, nor think about lunch, so he grabs what he can, and when the weekend finally arrives, he's run down, grumpy and not in the mood to face the gym.

Sunday evening means Monday morning is looming.

Realising he hasn't worked out in a week; George knows his previous efforts have been wasted and pointless. He wants to do something good for himself, but he believes he's messed up now, so quits going to the gym (but still keeps the membership going at £29.99 a month). The takeaways also creep back in and three and a half weeks after he started, George has stopped and feels worse than ever, as the lack of action has now coupled with self-administered guilt making him feel like a fraud and a failure.

All this just reinforces what George has heard since school and believed ever since:

That fitness is something *other people* do.

...But it doesn't have to be that way, I promise.

Working with more than 1,400 clients, all around the world, George's story is based on a multitude of tales, all along these lines.

I get it. Even with the pandemic, modern life is still really busy in many ways; what compounds this is, in recent years, the glorification of busy.

"How are you?"

"Busy!"

"Nice!"

Please, let's all work on stopping this. 'Busy' doesn't need to be worn as a badge of honour, and just because you're bust doesn't mean you're actually getting anything useful done.

The two other factors keeping George stuck are absolutely nothing to do with him.

Firstly, pressures to look, live, act, talk, BE a *certain way*

Secondly, the Fitness-sodding-Industry making everything far more complicated than it needs to be

Let's look at those. While it may be easy to blame social media, that isn't the problem as such. Social media is just the facilitator. A faster-and-more-addictive-every-year way to compare yourself.

That's what part of the problem is here, but comparing yourself and feeling lacking or insecure has been around well, forever. I'm not a big Bible fan, but isn't one of the 10 commandments: *Thou shalt not covet thy neighbour's ass?* (Stop making up your own jokes.)

Probably the best advice in that book. That and do not kill people. Try not to do that either.

So, if we agree it's in human nature to compare ourselves a little bit, and that actually, if you can take it with a pinch of salt and keep it at arm's length (and any other metaphors you fancy), then comparison *can* be useful...

Then we call it *inspiration*.

When you're inspired by someone, you might want to emulate them or their achievements in some way, that means you've experienced it as a force for good and are taking action (or planning to, soon) - lovely!

Being inspired by someone is a beautiful thing, and I have grown and developed and progressed most of all by maneuvering myself to be around amazing people from whom I can learn (and avoid the mistakes they made before me).

But when we compare ourselves - especially to the shiny, polished, not-really-real-but-we've-all-stuck-a-filter-on-a-selfie-haven't-we - world on social media, we start to ladle in guilt, sometimes shame too. We beat ourselves up with the word 'should' and so it feels like everyone else is having fun while we're eating crap, have an achy lower back and are watching a crappy sitcom that we think we might have already seen anyway.

Whether or not you buy into there being more pressure on the gay community to look a certain way for each other (and I'll discuss this more later), we also do it for the outside world. When coming to terms with my sexuality, I used to think that if I built up my body then I could 'pass' for straight (though I'm yet to be set an exam on this).

My homosexual desire to look as heterosexual as possible also added internal pressure. At one point, I remembering thinking: well, if I *have* to be gay, at least I won't be one of *those* gays… Whatever that means. I hate that I thought this previously; one of the joys of what I do now is how it brings me into contact with the whole spectrum of the amazing, inspiring LGBTQ+ community.

Looking back, 20-year-old Matt was scared, confused and unsure how he would ever fit in to a community of which he had very little experience… I had much more experience with straight people, hence my desire back then to be part of their world. (Yes, that is a Little Mermaid reference.)

The good news is, I have lots of different ways to help you with this in the section on Mindset.

Before that, let's examine the other sometimes-negative force at work here: the Fitness Industry overcomplicating things.

"You need to go Keto!"

"No, you need to go Paleo!!"

"Screw that, you need to be fasting for 19 and half minutes every three hours, and then for 24- and three-quarter minutes every five hours for the subsequent 21 hours!!!"

"No, you just need to give up sugar and do fasted workouts!!!!!"

"If you're not starting your day with 170mls of apple cider vinegar, you may as well be mainlining heroin - you're not a heroin addict, ARE YOU?!?!?!?!"

I could go on... (it *is* fun to write those sorts of things, but I'll stop at five of them).

But being obsessed with the new and the complicated is a major flaw in the fitness industry.

While the above methods might work for some people, most of us just need a sensible, sustainable way forward. This isn't to say I haven't fallen for things like this in the past.

In 2011, I paid for some EXTORTIONATELY expensive personal training for six weeks at a very unfriendly gym which recommended - I shit you not - taking 5 capsules of BCAA powder (bits of protein, don't worry about the detail) *in between sets in my workouts!* That meant upwards of 60 capsules a workout! I'd try to swallow them with minimal water so I didn't have it sloshing about in my stomach, meaning invariably a tablet or two would get stuck in my throat, so when I coughed, I exhaled a mysterious mist, like a confused and asthmatic dragon.

It did nothing for my training or progress in the short term, but in the long term... Well, of course it did nothing either. It was a ridiculous thing to do, and I know better now, but at the time, at the start of my fitness career, I just assumed that I should defer my knowledge to anyone who was older or stronger than I was.

The best thing about that nonsensical action was that it was *so* nonsensical, it helped me craft what Fitter Confident You is and does – i.e., the 180 degrees opposite of that.

You don't need any supplements (more on Nutrition in the section on the basics), especially not when starting out, but this is a common misconception and barrier that people put up themselves (they don't put it *up* themselves, they... oh, you know what I mean). So many beginners have actually held off beginning, because they believe they don't have the 'right' shoes, workout gear, supplements, gym membership, plan etc.

I'm here to show you that you don't need any of that. I think we've all put up barriers previously when starting something unknown, something we're nervous about. These barriers mean we delay getting started. A small, rational voice inside might be saying "we don't need to buy new trainers, we can go to that exercise class today!", but if another voice is saying "what if I don't know what to do in the class and people look at me", the voice of uncertainty often wins.

I know you've tried all sorts of needlessly complicated fitnesses and nutritionisms (I think those are the technical terms) which never quite stuck. Fitter Confident You is about bringing it back to basics, helping you build a fitness and well-being routine that suits you and fits your life and schedule (more on this when we get to workouts), one that never feels too much, overwhelming or not possible... But that helps you feel amazing, inside and out. That boosts your confidence and helps you absolutely LOVE who you see in the mirror, which you deserve more than pretty much anything else in life.

You'll find so many lovely stories from the Fitter Confident Youniverse, all the way through this book; they're here to inspire, encourage, and lift you up, but most of all, show you that anyone can do this. Anyone.

It's about reminding you that baby steps are always the best steps - they'll always get you where you want to go, but never feel off-putting.

It's about showing you it can be fun too! I know that might seem a million miles away to some of you right now, but I promise it can be.

Also, you're not lazy; allow me to explain:

Consider the thing you love doing the most in the world - this can be absolutely anything. When the time comes to do that, you don't delay, it just happens. You plan for it. You block out time in your diary. You don't let anything (or anyone) get in the way of you doing your favourite thing because - durrr - it's your favourite thing! When things are fun and enjoyable, we make time for them... You can probably see the segue coming here a mile off. So, you're not lazy around exercise, you just haven't had a plan built around YOUR needs, drivers and goals.

And most of all, that fitness, wellbeing, health - however you want to think of it - is absolutely, 100%, undeniably and irrefutably for you. For me. For him. For her. For them. For EVERYONE.

And I'm so excited to bring this all to life for you.

Shall we get started?

Matt Boyles

FIRSTLY, WHAT'S THE POINT OF LGBTQ-SPECIFIC TRAINING?

THE OBVIOUS ANSWER IS THAT WE'RE DIFFERENT. Only, of course, we're not.

But at the same time... we are.

Before you throw this book in the bin due to the author contradicting himself, please give me a chance to elaborate.

Physically, we're the same - we're all very much the same! There are some differences on a hormonal level between male, female, and non-binary bodies, but all bodies obey the laws of thermodynamics, all bodies convert food into energy that allows them to do... whatever they want to do each day. All bodies can get stronger, leaner, faster, jump higher and just do more stuff.

In my posts, I talk about who I specifically help and love to work with - the LGBTQ+ community - but lots of people who choose to comment on them seem to willfully misunderstand this and use it as a reason to bring out their inner troll.

Straight men 'hilariously' tagging their friends on my ads saying "Oi Smithy, this is what you need crying laughing emoji, crying laughing emoji, crying laughing emoji crying laughing emoji" etc. is always a real rib-tickler. Even worse is the out and out homophobic abuse.

I'm not telling you this for sympathy, I'm telling you this because it perfectly explains WHY we need community-specific services.

That an advert they could just scroll past elicits a "I must comment and tell this stranger why they're bad" response speaks volumes - we're equal on paper, but not in spirit, not in the streets, not online and certainly not in many, many other countries.

Rightly, the physical training elements of Fitter Confident You are the same for my clients as they would be for anyone else - and the FCY approach is all about simplifying things, which is why it works so well. However, it's the other components that make it relevant and built around our needs.

Private groups - safe spaces - where people can truly, finally, be themselves. Where questions can be asked without any fear of judgement. Where partners, boyfriends, husbands can be mentioned without members having to forcibly 'out' themselves into the unknown. Where there is empathy - because I've been there; because the FCY Client Success Coach David has also been there. To deeply understand what it feels like to walk into a gym and not feel like you belong and then to learn that you never need step foot in a gym again to make the progress you deserve.

To feel listened to, understood and truly heard... that's the power and gift of working with my community, and I'm so grateful I chose to go all in and support us with my whole chest.

So no, Fitter Confident You doesn't create workouts that are designed for gay men, or bisexual women, or trans men; it offers support and a truly tailored approach for each person based on their unique starting point, set-up and goals.

Starting a workout routine can feel hard enough already, without the added pressure of seemingly hyper-masculine environments and straight trainers who might not get why you don't feel 100% comfortable in a gym. This book is about you finding your own way, helping you write the future you want and doing it all on your terms.

LET'S BEGIN WITH THE BASICS

"I DON'T KNOW WHERE TO START."

And that's ok.

No one is expecting you to know precisely what to do to get started and find a way forward that you can stick to (apart from you and the weird expectations you put on yourself - stop that!).

This section will walk you, step-by-step, through the best ways (yes, multiple) to begin with some of this lovely fitnessy and wellbeing stuff I keep talking about.

I hope you're already starting to see that it doesn't need to be difficult, challenging, full-on or any adjective that just means 'a bit much'.

For everyone coming from a standing start, the best - and, yes, sometimes hardest - thing is to remove any notion of this being a quick fix. Starving yourself to fit into a pair of swimming shorts because you think you need to look a certain way for your holiday is a one-way ticket to unhappiness.

Repeat after me:

This is not a quick fix.

This is not about getting a six pack in a month.

This is not about doing extreme things for fast results that you only endure (rather than enjoy) and that causes misery, after which, you end up bouncing back to where you are now (or past it).

If you want that, this is not the book for you - I know, possibly too late to be warning you, but hey-ho.

Whatever you think at the moment, you CAN find the joy, the fun, the pleasure in getting into a routine with your health and fitness, and when you do and realise things are starting to fall into place, it's just *chef's kiss*, *100*, *heart eyes* or any other super happy feel-good emoji you fancy.

So, we're changing your brief that this isn't an 'overnight-transformation-from-lipo' situation - awesome.

Now, let's get physical...ly active (to avoid being sued by the writer of a similarly-named song!).

I recommend adding in just one new thing a week. Whatever you say or think, humans are actually terrible at multitasking, and some studies have indicated that trying to multitask is actually making us less adept at all of our tasks.

If you haven't done anything structured for a long time, start with walking. I know you know this, but if you're not doing it, then it needs re-stating. Choose a time and aim to go for a 10-minute walk for four days out of the next seven.

There's a great app called Streaks which has helped lots of clients build habits, as it encourages you to keep the streak (of whatever you're doing) going. Has anyone used Streaks to encourage regular streaking? Almost certainly.

Did you get those walks done - brilliant! Doesn't seem like much? Well, it's 4,000,000%* more than you did the week before, so I'd say that's progress AND I'd say it's worth celebrating.

*That number is correct because science + maths.

This is the second thing to start doing: acknowledging and celebrating the wins and ways you're progressing. No one else is going to do it for you, so even if you take a moment to privately celebrate, please do so. The more little boosts like these that you have through your week, the happier you're going to feel about what you're doing AND the more motivated you're going to feel to keep it all going.

Better still is if you can find ways to share it publicly too - not because we need social validation of what we're doing - that comes from within - but because you'll be passing on good energy and inspiring people around you, in all sorts of different ways.

The next habit to add in, is to check your water intake.

Under 2.5 litres a day? Slowly and steadily nudge it up. Think of water as the oil in an engine, it just makes everything work more smoothly and efficiently, while also boosting mental acuity, focus and recovery from your walks.

Right, you're two weeks in, you're doing your four walks a week - which, because you've got a bit fitter, you've started to make slightly longer - plus you're drinking a bit more water. Well done!

Let's add in a little bit of strength work. 10 push-ups please - this and hundreds of other explainer videos are available on my YouTube channel;

https://www.youtube.com/c/FitterConfidentYou.

Start by doing them on the three days you're not walking at first. On your knees is great, and split them up as needed too, but this will help you use your muscles in different ways now, specifically helping you build upper body strength and muscle.

Why are we doing this? Building strength is the most important thing we can do for our health and future happiness.

When you can lift a box onto a high shelf without any worry of your back going, when you can run for the bus and make it, when you can help a friend move a bed and barely break a sweat, life just flows more easily. So, start to get your push-ups done - and in this instance, you'll be surprised at how quickly you progress with this - you'll be doing them on your toes and daily in no time!

Now let's think about food.

Mmmm, custard doughnuts...

Not like that! But also, *yes like that!*

Food is a joy and I want you to go on enjoying it. I don't want you to create any strange rules or develop any unhealthy relationships with it, as, trust me, it's always going to be around, so the more you get on with it, the easier every day is.

But *thinking about food* really is the cornerstone to mastering your relationship with it.

Why?

Because so many of us just... don't. I know you're busy, I know you have work, friends, family, maybe a relationship, hobbies and more to juggle, but starting to be a bit more mindful about your food choices makes SUCH a difference.

That doesn't mean you have to track every calorie in every meal and know the precise nutritional breakdown of what's in your sandwich - that will most likely *lead* to a nutritional breakdown, and we definitely don't want that.

Start with your hunger cues. When you feel hungry, question if you really are hungry - sometimes this is easy (at least logically easier). Imagine, you've just had dinner and had the few extra potatoes that were staring at you, fine.

You clear up, sit down to watch TV and then five minutes later you're 'hungry'.

We can all agree you're not really hungry, but you've created a scenario with triggers and cues that mean the obvious next step is to get a pack of biscuits... because it's what you always do.

But just because you've always done something doesn't mean it's right for you.

This is not to blame or shame you (and I'll say this repeatedly through the book); if you want the biscuits, please eat them with my blessing.

But - and this is where the 'being a bit more mindful' part comes in - if you know there's about 100 calories in each biscuit (a handy rule of thumb), then 3 of those over the course of the evening could be the reason you're not losing weight - if that's your goal.

You may not even know you do this yet. There used to be a TV show called *Secret Eaters* where couples or families were trying to lose weight but it wasn't happening for them, despite their best efforts.

The show then set up cameras in their house - not hidden, they consented to this - and always picked up the extra food they were eating, without really being aware of it. Not sleep-eating (although having had some strange adventures while asleep myself, I can believe it's real) just normal, awake, finding food and then eating it food consumption. Because it was outside the usual times of breakfast, lunch and dinner, it just didn't register with them.

If you live with someone, you might want to ask them if they've spotted you doing any secret eating - or in-public eating that you're also not clocking.

And that's it.

Yes, really. That's what I would suggest to help you get moving, if you're coming from a standing start:

- Start walking regularly and intentionally
- Check your water consumption and steadily increase if needed
- Begin some regular mini home workouts - push-ups, squats, a few of each is all you need at the start
- There are some easy, 12-minute follow-along workouts on my YouTube channel you might like to try - *The 12 Minute Fix*
- Look at what you're eating and honestly see if it could be adjusted - asking a friend for input if necessary

Start this, and I guarantee, after a couple of weeks, you'll notice three things:

1. Your physicality will change - for the better; you'll feel fitter, stronger, lighter, have more energy, all good things
2. You'll start naturally doing a bit more - it's human nature to do so. Maybe you'll extend your walks, or do more of them. When you realise you can do all 10 push-ups on your knees without stopping you'll try one on your toes
3. The positive ripple effect will start to spread to other parts of your life - setting better boundaries in your relationships, finding you have more confidence at work

4. Some of the people in your life will notice too - again, we don't do it for external validation, but if it happens, we say 'thank you!'

All of which is absolutely flipping beautiful!

And if you pause or your burgeoning rhythm gets interrupted? Remember this, it's NOT ruined, it's just a blip. Get back to it when you can, and ask for help when you need it.

Fitter Confident You Client Stories: Matt Cunnington

What I was doing before

Before joining the Fitter Confident Youniverse, I didn't really have a routine of any kind. I worked a high-pressured job with tight deadlines. I had to visit more than 60 different towns and cities every six months, staying in hotels five nights a week, living on restaurant food and take outs and propping up the hotel bar.

My role involved coaching and training large teams on a daily basis and I threw myself into it. On the weekends and when I wasn't working, I'd release the tension by partying my free time away, living on cigarette fumes and very little sleep. Looking back now, I was rarely sober in my free time. I was so invested in supporting people at work, but I was failing to pay attention to my needs.

Instead, I was burning the candle at both ends and leading a hedonistic lifestyle. On the surface I looked happy and I always had a smile on my face, but in reality, I was depressed and on the verge of breaking down.

As a result, I was seeking comfort in things that weren't that great for me. I used cigarettes, alcohol, hook-ups and sugar... So much sugar, anything with an instant reward.

I was diagnosed with osteoporosis in 2013 after breaking my hip. It means my bones are fragile and more likely to break and could result in me being in a wheelchair later in life, but I did nothing to strengthen my bones to avoid that from happening. I stuck my head in the sand and pretended it wasn't happening.

When lockdown hit, I went into a crisis. My mental health declined day-by-day. The partying stopped because it had to and anxiety crept in. I had zero self-esteem and body confidence.

I didn't know who I was and I weighed just under 8 stone. I had no routines that protected my wellbeing. Plus, I didn't know how or where to start.

Changing routines

Changing my entire routine was a gradual process and happened over two years. First, I left London and moved back with my parents - there's so much to be said for having a great support network around you, whoever that may be.

Next came food. Simply put, just eating three meals a day. Then I started meditation, mindfulness techniques and light exercise to improve my mental health. Until this point, I'd always avoided exercise, I hated it. But... I didn't like who I was anymore. I knew I had to do something for me, something new, challenging, and healthy. So, I contacted Matt and got enrolled.

I bought weights and started on three home workouts a week, eventually moving up to four. I built exercise into my working day so I'd start in the evening after work. At first, I wasn't enjoying it anywhere near as much as I do now so I held myself accountable by inviting friends along to join me virtually over webcam and including my dad in the routines.

I took photos each month as I found motivation in the progress I was seeing. I aimed to beat my previous personal bests as much as I could - mainly so I could celebrate with Matt in our regular catch ups - and over time, I started to feel better about myself each day.

Before I started exercising, I was terrified of falling over in case I broke something. I felt weak and vulnerable. A few months into working with Matt, I fell down the stairs and I'll never forget how I felt when I caught myself. My arms were strong and supported my body weight out and I regained my balance.

It was then I realised I'd made a really positive change. My balance had improved, my weight was increasing, I liked what I saw in the mirror and most importantly to me, I could control my future. I don't need to give up and accept that my bones will get weaker over time. I can fight it by getting stronger. It isn't always easy. I don't always hit my target of 4 workouts a week and It's taken me a while to learn that that's ok, I just go again next time.

The future

Next, I'll be leaving the UK for 6 months to travel through Central America and then to live in Costa Rica. I recently visited and fell in love with the place. It was a true adventure holiday, I went kayaking, horse riding, scuba diving - all things I'd never felt I was capable of before.

I took my top off on the beach and was happy to have my photo taken - another first! I've taken a sabbatical from work and my flights are booked. As the months have gone on I felt better about myself and more confident in my own skin. I've regained my sense of adventure and know that, with patience and time, I can achieve what I want if I put my mind to it.

MINDSET

 "Whether you think you can or you can't, you're right."

OK, OK, I APPRECIATE THIS SOUNDS LIKE ONE OF those glib, see-it-on-Instagram quotes that people churn out... But self-belief (even a really small amount at the start) is the difference between making the progress you want and staying stuck.

That's why I said 'even a really small amount', because this isn't a binary situation of either having self-belief or not. It's instead a spectrum - a sliding scale - on which all of us exist, moving up and feeling a bit more confident and inspired, and sometimes slipping down a bit, which is part of the process.

The binary, 'on/off', 'have/don't have' way of thinking is one of the big causes of people feeling stuck. I've heard from countless people who are waiting for the moment when they're confident enough to do something.

"I'll start working out when I've lost 5kg."

"I'll book that holiday when I'm feeling more body confident."

"I'll be happy when I can fit into 34" jeans."

Allow me to absolutely, categorically, definitely and 100% confirm that those feelings of confidence and happiness do not come from waiting for them.

To paraphrase Oliver Burkeman in his brilliant book 'Four Thousand Weeks':

This future-facing way of living - *when* I achieve a certain thing I'll *finally* be happy and can relax as I will have *mastered* my life - means you'll never be fulfilled, as you're treating the present as a path to a superior future, so the present will *never* feel satisfying.

Even if you do hit those goals and somehow feel you've got everything under control, there will always be something else placed ahead of you that will seem more appealing.

The only way we feel better and improve what we want to improve, is by taking action.

That may instantly have sent you back into thinking in the binary way:

"I have to overhaul my life, I have to exercise for at least an hour, five days a week, I have to give up all the foods I like..."

Take a breath, it's ok. That's not the way either!

That might have been how you tried to do it before, but I know it didn't stick, because it wasn't enjoyable, it took over your life and was always front of mind - *can I have that food? How many calories will this run burn off? I shouldn't have that glass of wine...*

Start small, start slow, build up ever so - ever so! - steadily, and it will never feel too much, it won't take over your life, you won't see food as something else to stress over and you WILL make the progress you're after.

Here are the key Fitter Confident You elements to making it all work for you - plus some practical tips to really make it stick.

1. Start very slowly and steadily so it never feels too much
2. Find ways to make it enjoyable
3. Get some accountability
4. Put some goals in place...
5. Work on getting more excited about *the journey* - celebrating the processes will help you stay the course far more than waiting... and waiting... and waiting for the end goals to be achieved
6. Dial into *everything* that's happening as a result of what you've started and celebrate every win and progress point along the way, especially the small ones
7. Find your tribe for extra support and encouragement
8. Realise that progress - fat loss, strength, fitness, muscle building - is NEVER linear, even though our brains tell us it should be
9. Unfollow people on social media who don't inspire you the right way

10. Remember 99.9% of social media is faked, or at least filtered and molded to be an exaggeration of the truth

11. You never need set foot in a gym or pay for a gym membership to make the progress you want

12. A little bit of planning goes a very long way - for example, scheduling workouts into your diary makes you and your brain start to see them as just as important as any other appointment (which they are!) so you'll make time for them too

13. You don't need to give up any of your favourite foods to make the progress you want to see

14. Take pics every four weeks - it might feel uncomfortable there and then, but soon you'll be happy you have a visual record of your progress

15. Your body is the least interesting thing about you... I know that sounds mean, allow me to explain: the less you focus on how you look and the more you focus on what you can do, the more inspired you will feel - as Judge Judy says *"beauty fades, dumb is forever"*

16. Most people start by focusing on what you want to lose - fat, reduce waist size, reduce a health risk - which will work for a bit, but focusing on what you have to gain (see below) is so much more fun, inspiring, exciting, and has proven to be so much more sustainable, time and again - and this is from firsthand experience and witnessing Fitter Confident You clients and the Fitter Confident You group members change their focus.

And now, a non-exhaustive (but still quite long!) list of what you have to gain from starting a bit of fitness...

1. Better sleep
2. More energy day-to-day
3. Better, more stable mood
4. Less instances of anxiety and depression
5. Better able to cope with stress
6. Greater self-love
7. Greater appreciation for what you can go on to achieve (i.e., motivation!)
8. Higher sex drive and higher testosterone
9. Lower cortisol levels (stress hormone)
10. Greater strength
11. Stronger back that can cope with anything
12. Stronger immune system
13. General all-over futureproofing!
14. Run faster
15. Run further
16. Jump higher
17. Do your favourite hobbies or sports for longer
18. Greater confidence to speak up at work
19. Greater ability to respect your own boundaries
20. Loving who you see in the mirror
21. Better balance (sounds a bit dry, but when you get older, being in your 70s and not falling over regularly is a really good thing)
22. Better coordination
23. Higher bone density - some HIV medication has been linked to a reduction in bone density, but resistance training (weight lifting, using TRX, resistance bands or bodyweight training) has been proven to counteract this
24. Inspire those around you that you know

25. Inspire those around you that you *don't* know.

To explain number 25 in a bit more detail…

One of my favourite things is how you'll start inspiring and lifting up those you know in your circle of friends, family, colleagues, and online. But even more excitingly…

Due to all the lovely ways in which you'll evolve, the positive ripple effect spreads out across the world. For example, you had a good workout with a friend, putting you in a better mood than if you hadn't exercised, so when you go to a coffee shop afterwards, you're feeling more confident and end up having a lovely chat with the guy who works there, who, unbeknownst to you, had just broken up with his boyfriend and was feeling a bit crap. You forget the conversation afterwards, but you lifted his spirits that day, and he is a bit more smiley to the customers after you… And so the goodness continues ever onwards.

Why is building a wellbeing routine we can stick to so important for the LGBTQ+ community?

How long have you got?!

Any minority is subject to pressures, situations, aggressions and trauma that our counterparts will never go through. They may hear and understand these, but they will never live it.

Growing up in the UK in the 1980s, the Conservative government of the time introduced a Local Government Act, within which was the now notorious Section 28, which forbade the 'promotion of homosexuality' in school.

This meant it couldn't be discussed by teachers in any way. It couldn't be presented as a normal way of life; it 'othered' everyone who wasn't straight. There were threats of prosecution to schools who did discuss or teach about LGBTQ+ life, and to a boy coming to terms with his sexuality, starting to realise he was different, it felt very strange to be at school but excluded in so many ways.

Sex education in general was perfunctory at best, but the only healthy relationship and way forward that was presented, was a man and a woman.

Just when young people should be supported and listened to, there was silence.

It also emboldened some pupils to use 'gay', 'fag' or 'that's gay' as an insult.

Couple this with the media presentation of gay people - either predatory or the harmless, sexless, camp man - and it's easy to see why so many people grow up confused, in denial and often with a combination of self-loathing (internalised) *and* externalised homophobia.

More than 30 years on, it turns out no one was prosecuted under Section 28, and the Baroness who brought it to parliament has offered a half-hearted apology:

"I'm sorry if anyone was hurt by it" - that *'if'* really sticks in the throat, doesn't it.

I'm grateful that my school was fairly supportive in some ways; there wasn't the extreme bullying that I've heard about happening elsewhere. However, Section 28 looming over us forced young people to 'in' themselves, forcing us to self-censor and modify who we were and how we acted and looked, for fear of standing out for the wrong reasons.

And the spectre of that era stays with many of us today. Feelings of inadequacy, not being good enough, being unsure, even now, how we should present ourselves - will the new people we meet today be hostile or accepting? When the rules and messages from the very top of society are that gay people are wrong, dangerous, other, it trickles down and legitimises those views in the street and online.

One workout won't undo years of discrimination, but the power of a bit of regular exercise - and any other things you do to help you feel better - is that it does remind you of your power.

Seeing, feeling, and just *knowing* that you're making progress can be the spark to help you stand a bit taller, make eye contact with a bit more confidence.

Part of it is realising you can rely on yourself that bit more, that you can make progress physically and emotionally too, which is tough to put into words as it really is a feeling, a sense of ownership and responsibility in your life.

It can also help you step away from any victim mentality you're holding onto - that realisation that no one is coming to save you. Yes, you can ask for help and support and guidance, but you have to decide to put one foot in front of the other, to commit to something really good for you, long term.

And when that happens, the snowball starts to grow and grow, and in the same way a rolling snowball gains size, speed and momentum, so you too will find it easier to stick to your routine, to make time for it, to make time for YOU and to make it happen each week.

I'm very happy to say that from what I see and hear from my younger relatives, the next generations are behaving differently. They're taking each other at face value and basing their opinions and relationships on who each of them are, not from a pre-disposed, inherited belief that some people aren't normal, which gives me hope that it will never be as bad for us again.

Fitter Confident You Client Stories: Kieran Moore

"Kieran Moore. Hero or villain?"

I'll never forget those words.

It was a sunny July afternoon. My first ever PE lesson in "Big School". I was there on an induction day to learn the ropes before making the leap the following September. And I was quite literally stepping up to bat.

I was a spindly kid with very little to recommend me athletically. My sporting achievements up to this point consisted of standing in goal while my brothers played football (since kicking the ball was generally beyond me), falling off a balance beam, and competing at a county event in a sack relay race (we came third).

And yet, a quiet hush fell across the gargantuan sports field as I picked up the rounders bat. All eyes were on me.

Sports just weren't my thing. I was a nerd - a textbook case. I'd worn glasses since preschool. I was one of the brightest in the school. Academia came easy to me. But I was awkward and scruffy and had haircuts in avant-garde styles that were never fashionable and never will be. Most of my classmates worked out I was gay before I did. I wished I'd listened when they told me so, instead of shrugging it off as baseless insults. I might have saved myself a few years…

And yet here we were – the rounders equivalent of the Olympics, football world cup or

Wimbledon – and it all depended on me.

I grew to hate PE lessons at school. I would get a note written whenever I could – particularly in the winter. My dad, who is quite sporty himself, eventually gave up and wrote me a note that said I had a leg injury and had to have at least a term (maybe more) off anything active. Every time I passed a PE teacher in the hall, I developed a limp. By the end of my school career, I simply bunked off entirely and went and sat at a nearby park for an hour. I had no interest in sport and sport (or at least PE lessons) had said "Thanks, but no thanks" on several occasions. It was a conscious uncoupling.

The warm air hung motionless and time stood still. If movie tropes were real, a crow would have called out ominously and my mother would have been weeping. "But he's only a child!" she'd have wailed.

After school I developed a love of food. But my culinary deities were less Egon Ronay and more Big Kev off the chip van. No food was left unfried and my brother and I invented a late-night version of a full English that would fell a rhinoceros. It's fair to say I put on weight.

It's also fair to say this suited me. As a young lad who didn't really want to be gay, being unattractive meant I didn't have to worry about a romantic relationship of any description so, the un-confrontable could go un-confronted.

As I made my way to the batting area, I considered where it had all gone wrong. My lack of sports confidence meant I'd hung back in the queue and with one ill-fated swing of a rounders bat I was about to ruin the next five years of my life.

Through most of my adulthood, sport and fitness had been a no-go. It was something other people did. I didn't understand runners at all. Why would you do that? What was the point?

That said, I remember one occasion where my brother and I decided we'd run a marathon.

We did one small jog around our local park, felt outrageously self-conscious and never did it again. I didn't really weigh myself but my waist size peaked at 44". Occasionally, my size would bother me. There was one afternoon where I hit a deep depression and saw something truly hideous in the mirror – none of my clothes could disguise how awful I looked and I refused to go out. But I saw it as my body, my choice and I was pragmatic about it all. I liked food and wanted to enjoy it. I also didn't want to confront my truth...

My team was currently drawing with the opposition. I was living every sports movie ever made. When Mr. Allen asked the ultimate question, "Kieran Moore, hero or villain?", he meant it.

There's only so long you can live a lie before it takes its toll and at age 40, I finally had to cough up and cross the bridge. I hit a period of depression and knew I had to get something off my chest. I finally told my friend I was gay. He was marvellous (and still is). And as I battled depression and tried to put together what was about to become my life something amazing happened. The weight I had been carrying started to fall away. I pounced on this and got a GP referral to my local gym. I loved it! The gym was my sanctuary and though it wasn't always easy to get through the door, once I did, I was in my own little world. I would make sure every session included a personal best – one extra rep here, two extra pounds lifted there – fitness suddenly became the place I got my wins and not my fails!

I gulped as the ball left the bowler's hand, closed my eyes and swung.

Over the next few years, I used the gym, a personal trainer and some of the most supportive people I've ever known to fight off a diabetes scare, hit my target weight and go from a size XXL to a small. But most importantly, I found myself and became happier, fitter and more confident. Sport and fitness made me the person I was supposed to be.

Who would have thought? And it still gives me wins to this day. Last year I completed my first marathon and this year, my second (knocking 25 minutes off my PB)! But above all this, and despite listing above all the people and places that helped, the biggest win is knowing that I did this. I made it happen. I backed myself, took a big swing and won.

So, on that fateful day was I a hero or a villain? In some ways, I don't think it really matters.

All I'll say is that if you swing big enough, you're bound to hit something. And I took a very big swing that day.

MY FITTER CONFIDENT STORY...

WHICH HAS BEEN PEPPERED THROUGHOUT THE book. But so you can see that anyone - anyone! - can do this, here's my journey from someone who was very not interested in fitness, sport and 'the like', to, well, someone whose life and path has been completely altered by it.

For the better!!! (Just to be clear - although it would be funny if you got to this point and I suddenly said STOP!)

This isn't a call to arms to get you to quit your job and become a Personal Trainer (though if you want to, go for it!) it's to show you what can happen when you begin to bet on yourself. Your journey will look completely different to mine, but there will be parallels and key lessons I can share from what got me to right here, right now: 2022, running a growing online fitness company, 41 years old, best strength and fitness of my life and heart-burstingly proud of what I do.

The biggest takeaway (apart from that biryani I had last week) is that everything you want - and lots you don't even know you want yet - is in reach.

Actually, there's another really big one:

Don't sweat it if you haven't figured it out yet, or feel you don't have a plan or goal or grand scheme. I'm not sure anyone does, not really, but you CAN get lots better at zeroing in on what lights you up - and as I get older, life becomes about stringing together more of those events that do just that.

Let's look at the key phases of my life:

0 - 3; The Baby Years

Unremarkable. Couldn't even conjugate verbs. Regular nappy-filler.

4 - 12; The Junior School Years

Did PE. Rounders, running, swimming, enforced rugby (not a fan). Was really good at skipping, but boys didn't do that after the age of 6, did they?! (Tell THAT to Crossfit!)

13 - 18; The Senior School Years

Bit of athletics, a few random other things. No real reason for any of the subjects I chose for A-Level - I didn't want to be a doctor, so I didn't have to do the sciences, so I just went with... 'things? Oh ok, Geography, Business Studies, German, and the VERY USEFUL General Studies.

On the very last day of school, I won the Headmaster's Prize, which was very nice of them, but was a bit 'well he was nice and well behaved and did some things but was never really outstanding in any particular field, but we should probably give him something, oh yes, this will do'. You can also file this under 'God loves a trier'.

But that was me then, and for quite a while after. Which is fine and I don't regret taking longer to find myself. I just wasn't ready back then. It's been amazing watching *Heartstopper* recently and seeing the growing acceptance of LGBTQ+ people from a younger age.

I wasn't bullied explicitly, but being naturally skinny and friends with lots of girls, I would sometimes hear "gay" thrown at me, as an insult... Which was funny at the time, as I was adamant, I wasn't...

19 - 22; The University Years

I 'studied' American Studies at Swansea University in South Wales. First time living away from home. Tentative steps to find out who I was, what I liked. Amazing year abroad in Long Beach in Southern California.

I was starting to realise those boys at school maybe knew I was gay before I did. I still dated girls for some of these years but was now meeting a few gay people, who at some points, I went out of my way to avoid, not wanting to be associated with them - I know, internalised homophobia and shame is an ugly weight around our necks.

It was while living in America that I went through a phase of writing BMM on my hand for a while:

Be More Masculine.

Where's the smack my head emoji when you need it?

This was how I thought I should 'present' to fit in, to be accepted, to make friends and move ahead. Really sad, actually, the more I think about it.

I joined a gym for the first time while in Long Beach and started buying Men's Health Magazine to learn what to do. The gym was in a giant blue pyramid, which was appealing. Oh, and I tried protein shakes for the first time too, and let me tell you, in 2001 they were revolting. You people trying them in 2022 for the first time, you don't know you're born!

Still no idea about what I wanted to do or who I was going to be when I grew up.

23 - 30; The Employed Years

After university, and not knowing what to do, I did some classic try-regular-work-for-the-first-time jobs - the best/worst being handing out samples of toilet roll, dressed as the now-extinct Charmin Bear (RIP).

However, this was the period of the most seismic change: I moved to London and came out to myself and to my new friends, bit by bit.

The best way to describe it was turning the page and starting a brand new page - heck, a whole new volume in the book of my life.

Coming out was the best and most important personal step I've ever taken. In many situations, while 'the grass is greener on the other side', there's sometimes a troll under the bridge... or a UKIP rally in the field when you get to it...

But coming out was the one situation when the grass really *was* greener, and it meant I started to find and connect with some of my best friends, whom I still treasure - Stephen, David, James - now I've typed them, they sound like fake names, but I can't help it if my friends' names are run-of-the-mill, trust me, they run VERY brilliant, gay mills.

This was also when I tried an outdoor bootcamp for the first time, which I credit with awakening my love of fitness.

While it wasn't what I wanted to do long-term, it started to introduce all the different ways you can do fitness and crucially, just how good it can feel.

I was outside, with nice people, getting fitter, faster, stronger, making progress, and something just clicked.

I was working in a marketing agency at the time and then joined a gym near the office, trying some of the PTs there, who I assumed knew what they were talking about as they were bigger than me. Looking back, they were fine - fairly traditional in approach, but I learned different skills and exercises from them and they inspired me to get into a rhythm.

Oh, I also ran the London marathon in 2007, without a specific training plan which... I do not advise! Sure, run the marathon, but get a proper plan in place beforehand!

31 - 36; The Traditional Personal Training Years

Why did I become a PT back then? Honestly?

Work in the marketing agency was really busy and marketing wasn't a passion, so it was to work in an industry I cared about... And also to be able to train myself more often!

Qualifying as a Personal Trainer and going self-employed was a shock and hard to swallow for a number of people in my life, and yes, previously I hadn't really stuck at things in the past, but I knew, *I just knew*, that this was what I really wanted to do, that it would make me happy and fulfilled...

And it was!

End of Book, thanks for reading!!!

No, wait, there's more! Becoming a PT, I knew I didn't want to work in a gym. The only other way I could conceive was being an outdoor PT, so that's what I did. Bought a small car, filled the boot with mats, dumbbells, TRX, kettlebells and started finding clients.

Working in the park was brilliant when the sun was out... less so when it was 1 degree, raining and you put your hand in dog poo (yes really, ick).

BUT I adored it. I was outside, I attracted amazing, lovely clients who were easy to always show up for - I'm still friends with lots of them now. Plus I was working in an industry I really did love and bonus on bonus, I DID have more time to workout. I started going more regularly, found a gym buddy and started seeing how to push myself a bit more.

Oh! And I also ran a company called Wireless Fitness for a few years, with my friend Dom. We used silent disco equipment to run fitness classes outside without disturbing people in the park – what's that you say? Ahead of its time? Oh, stop!

We had some adventures with it and even went on Dragon's Den to raise money to create a Wireless Fitness app, but I don't like to talk about it... Just kidding, buy me a protein shake and I'll tell you all the goss from behind the scenes!

37 - 41 (now!); The Fitter Confident You Years.

I had loved my time training people in the park, but after six years, had an itch to do something new. It wasn't that I had gone off fitness, I just felt I could be doing more, learning and growing more.

Seeing the rise of online trainers around the world, I was inspired... But also thought I could do something a bit more specialised and a bit more special.

The youniverse aligned and I found an amazing training course designed specifically to teach face-to-face PTs how to become online PTs... and that was the catalyst for these years of adventure and growth.

I reckon you know the rest really, but taking the fork in the road that meant I moved online and created Fitter Confident You was hands down the best decision I've ever made. And heck! Hands up too!

Reflecting for a moment, and being very much a people person, one of the most amazing elements of the Fitter Confident Youniverse, is the number of amazing, brilliant, hilarious, kind, warm, welcoming and truly inspiring people I've had the honour of getting to know, whether we worked together 121 or just via the different online groups I've set up.

A huge thank you to all of you. This might feel like something you'd put at the end of the book, but I've discovered I quite like confounding expectations!

So, I'm quite literally here, typing my life story as it happens - very meta! What will happen next? Maybe I should write it and find out.

That sounds like one of those "hilarious" jokes, but the older I get, the more I see we have the power to write our story. We don't have to read other people's and follow their adventures, we get to have adventures of our own!

Only this morning, I was watching some brilliant training on mindset, that said how we're dragging around a wheelie-bag full of other people's hopes, opinions, beliefs, experiences and thoughts... And that it's ok to start taking them out, so we only have space for our own. Which I thought was a brilliant metaphor - if we have to pull a wheelie-bag of stuff, it might as well be ours!

Fitter Confident You Client Stories: Bill Gallagher

My history, before working with Matt...I was significantly obese throughout childhood and into my late 30s. When the scales hit 19 stone (266 pounds), I realised I needed to take action. I had been on countless diets – with little or no success. A friend persuaded me to join a gym.

The concept of a gym terrified me – but working on the principle of no pain = no gain, I took the plunge. This was the first time in my life that I had taken any exercise. I also concentrated on changing my diet.

The efforts paid off and I got down to a weight I was comfortable with after two years (I lost 90 pounds).

During these two years, the changes to my eating behaviour became second nature, and I realised I could continue to do this without much effort. But I could not get into the mindset of taking regular exercise – so I stopped going to the gym. I tried several times to restart at the gym, but this always stopped after a few weeks.

Working with Matt...

Roll forward 15 years or so and we find ourselves at the start of a pandemic and in a lockdown.

The good news is that I had maintained the same weight. This was achieved through a balanced approach to calories. But my only regular exercise was walking to and from the Tube on my daily commute. The enforced working from home took away this little bit of exercise.

Worried that this would lead to weight gain, I contacted Matt. I wanted to have a few exercises I could do at home.

Honestly, I had low expectations! I had tried and failed to get back into the habit of taking exercise so many times before.

But something clicked. Two years later I am taking regular exercise – and really enjoying it. I am in the best shape I have ever been (physically and mentally).

My journey since I started working with Matt...

I started working out from home, following a 12-week programme set by Matt. I enjoyed it and started to see some positive changes.

However, I still had my low expectations. Based on my previous pattern of experience I did not believe I would stick to the exercises in the long term. A lot of Matt's work is focussed on challenging expectations and patterns of behaviour.

For me, this is the biggest difference between Matt and other personal trainers. He helped me realise that I could change my mindset and that I was not doomed to fail.

I had a lightbulb moment. I realised that I had thought of exercise as a means to an end. 15 years ago, I started to go to the gym to get to a target weight. After hitting the target, I saw no continued need for the gym. I viewed it as a temporary effort needed to achieve a goal.

Matt successfully challenged my perceptions. I realised that I enjoyed taking exercise – so why would I stop something that I enjoyed? I also enjoy the physical and mental changes this brought (being stronger, having fewer aches and pains, losing a few inches around the waist and generally feeling more confident).

My biggest learning…

In my entire journey (initially through changing my eating habits and latterly getting into a regular exercise routine), I have had one major learning: our relationship with diet and exercise is formed in childhood – being influenced by the parents, caregivers, schools, etc. Sometimes we end up with a "disordered relationship" with food and/or exercise.

In a perfect world, children would learn a balanced approach to diet and exercise. But there are many examples of when this does not happen. With food, for example, parents sometimes use it to reward or to punish (e.g. 'you can have a biscuit if you finish your homework').

Fitness can follow a similar pattern. I always thought that fitness was for other people, but not for me.

This view was massively influenced by the attitudes of my parents and my reaction to school gym classes. This was formed in childhood and stayed – largely unchallenged – until recently.

Therefore, my biggest learning is that as a 'grown-up' I can take ownership of my relationship with diet and exercise. I do not need to repeat the patterns of my childhood.

SELF-LIMITING BELIEFS (AND KIND WAYS ROUND THEM)

ALL BELIEFS ARE SELF-LIMITING IN SOME WAY, because if you believe one thing, it means you're limiting what else you could believe in... Believe me!

But by saying 'Self-limiting beliefs', we all know what I'm about to talk about. So, let's crack on and let's see if I can't just help you understand yourself a bit more and see through some of these SLBs that have been holding you back...

I don't have the time

These aren't necessarily in the order of how often I hear them, but this one does come up fairly regularly. Because our days are portioned up into hours, and because PT sessions have traditionally been portioned up into hours... And even because our school PE sessions were - that's right! - portioned up into hours (or two hours!), it's understandable why so many people believe they need to commit to at least an hour for exercise to be worthwhile.

And if that's true, then you've also got the time getting to the gym, getting changed, warming up, the workout itself, chatting with your Gym Crush™, getting changed and showered, perusing the 'healthy snacks' vending machine, getting home or back to work... and that could be two hours out of your day.

So it's no wonder that can seem a bit off-putting.

But the thing is, it's not true. I promise it doesn't have to be like that.

For the quickest of all, home workouts require no commute, you can already be changed and ready, a warm-up can be done in 5 minutes, and 15 minutes later, you can be done and back at your desk (you can shower in the evening, they can't smell you on Zoom! (yet!)). 20ish minutes and you've done something SO good for you, your day and your future.

Does that now seem doable? Awesome. If you're starting out, two or three of those a week is all you need to make a difference to how you feel, your energy levels and your fitness and strength.

I don't have any motivation

I could write a whole book on this (and shhhh, don't tell anyone, I've actually sketched an outline for Book Two and it's all about Motivation!) but ok, THIS I do hear all the time, and yes, some level of motivation is needed, as all the knowledge in the world is completely pointless if you don't do something with it.

Here's what to do:

First off, grab a pen and paper and write down what you would do if you did have the motivation. These could be huge or tiny, but capture all the possibilities on that sheet of paper.

What's on it? Go to the gym before work? Go for a walk in your lunch break? Book swimming lessons this weekend? Get off the bus two stops earlier two nights a week? Prep some food?

Now you can see what you want to do, you can come up with practical solutions to make them happen and fit them into your week.

Often, the big realisation is simply that you're feeling tired, run down and just lacking the physical energy to do these. If that's the case, you can try a few things:

- Look at improving your sleep - even small changes add up to help you feel more rested - reducing caffeine, trying black-out blinds and avoiding screens and work emails before bed can all make a difference
- Are you hydrated enough? We feel sluggish mentally and physically when we're not drinking enough water, when did you last have a glass?
- You may be surprised that even a little bit of exercise can give you more energy, both straight afterwards and the next day. Bodies generally respond to movement, so the more you use your body, the easier

everything works and so the easier it is to *keep* using your body

I do appreciate those first steps might feel like the toughest. Newton's First Law of Motion states that an object at rest will stay at rest unless additional forces act on it - equally, an object in motion will stay in motion unless something acts on it, so yes, the inertia you feel at the moment IS real, but not insurmountable.

Another great way to beat the motivation blues to find your tribe. Find your best cheerleaders to support and encourage you - and for you to do the same to them, which is just as motivating.

It's why I created the free FCY Facebook Group (search for 'Online Personal Training - Fitter Confident You' on Facebook to join), which is an amazing resource designed to inspire, connect, motivate and encourage - all of which it does on a daily basis, to more than 5,000 members, all around the world!

I don't like exercise / I don't like the gym

Then I can't help... Only joking! I fully understand that not everyone will be as into the ol' fitness as I am, and that's fine. A world of me's would be... a lot.

What I've found when people say they don't like exercise is, 9 times out of 10, what they don't like is the idea of exercise OR the memory of it.

PE lessons at school were quite stressful for many of us - having an inkling we were gay, bi or trans - different in any way - around the same time only added to the pressures we felt. So it's unsurprising that for many of us, walking into a gym can elicit a deep, almost primal reaction.

If this is the case, starting with home workouts and learning how to exercise in the privacy of your own home or garden is a great way forward. There's no one else there to compare yourself to, you don't have to smell the same mass market toilet-cleaner which takes you back to school changing rooms and there's no pressure to stop using a piece of equipment because someone else is waiting.

Home workouts are also great because they reduce the commuting time to zero - just pop into your spare room and there you are - this also helps reduce the friction and resistance at getting a workout done.

I don't want to change what I'm eating

Guess what? You don't have to!

Well, if you subscribe to the old-fashioned diet-based ways of doing things (booooo! Don't do that!) then sure, cut out your favourite foods, give up wine, cut out caffeine, avoid pizza, forsake ice-cream and eat only lettuce and Ryvita for three months, but that route isn't sustainable and leads to really unpleasant withdrawal headaches!

So work *with* your human nature as opposed to against it.

If I said to you: *don't think about or eat any biscuits for six weeks*, I know for a fact you are now thinking about biscuits, and a small part of your brain is saying *oooh, aren't garibaldis nice*, and, *ooh yes, we've worked hard today, I wonder if there are any of those nice pink wafers in the house...*

It's just how we're wired.

STOP THINKING ABOUT JENNIFER LOPEZ RIDING A 30 FOOT HIGH PENGUIN!

We both know what you're thinking about now - me too, what an image!

So, as opposed to giving up any of your favourite foods and as opposed to going on a ridiculously restrictive diet, what Fitter Confident You teaches is how it all works.

We pull back the curtain on how nutrition works, tailor it to how it works specifically for you and then give you swaps, suggestions and strategies for how to stick to it, with the kindness and breathing space we all need.

I tried before and it didn't work

Ok, lots I can help you with here, but the answer will be there in whatever data/info you can tell me - you might secretly or subconsciously know it already.

THERE'S a great expression relevant here which is usually quoted as:

Success leaves clues

But we can flip it to:

Mistakes leave clues

What did you do last time?

Was it personalised?

Was it too much?

Was it too little?

Was it right for you?

Was it right for your goals?

Was it right for your schedule?

How long did you stick at it?

Did you have any support or accountability?

What did the nutrition coaching require of you?

Did you work hard enough?

Did you work too hard?

If you give me - or sometimes even just an impartial observer - the answers to some of these, I'll be able to figure out why it didn't happen for you last time.

I say 'impartial observer' as your partner or best friend may not tell you the truth - they love you and want the best for you and don't want to hurt your feelings, so will say "sure babe, you did give that last plan a chance..." - because in their mind, that's kinder - Instead of rationally examining what you tried and looking at logical reasons why you didn't make the progress you were after.

My body doesn't respond

Time for some tough love.

Your body *does* respond to stimuli, but for all manner of reasons (some listed above), it hasn't responded to what you've done before.

All bodies obey the laws of thermodynamics relative to energy, food and movement. If you stick to a kind, empathetic plan you start to enjoy, change WILL happen.

Another problem linked with this is focusing too much (or entirely!) on one metric - in most cases, this is usually weight loss - i.e., what the scales say.

When you focus on one metric, you miss all the other amazing things that are happening, and *those* go a long way to keep you excited and motivated about what you're doing. And if you're excited and motivated, then you keep doing what you're doing...

And if you keep doing what you're doing your body will respond - to use a double negative, it can't *not* respond.

So keep going, and celebrate and appreciate ALL the amazing wins and progress and developments that happen along the way.

Every week in the private Facebook group just for FCY clients, we have #WINSday; a chance for all the clients to share and celebrate their wins and learnings and progress made. Every week it's a wonderful and uplifting collection of gems that inspire, encourage and help to raise all of us up. (It also sounds like someone with a South African accent saying 'Wednesday', and we run it every Wednesday - double whammy!).

My Metabolism has slowed down

This has become a catch-all explanation for progress not being made, but it really isn't to blame.

There are three times in your life when your metabolism noticeably slows:

1. After the first 12 months of your life
2. When you stop growing, around age 20
3. In your 70s

But for the majority of us, for the 50 years between 20 and 70, your metabolism only slows a little bit. The reason most people don't lose weight during that time is that they're eating more than they need.

Again, this is never to blame or shame you, just to give you the science and facts to help you make sustainable, consistent changes you can stick to.

I feel intimidated by it all

I get that. I used to feel that way. So I've been collating a growing list of ways to build your GYMFIDENCE, which is coming up soon in its own chapter, as it's so big!

I don't know where to start / I don't know what works for me

My mission is to help as many LGBTQ+ people as possible, so go back to this chapter and see which bits are relevant to your journey.

I don't want to be shouted at or shamed by a PT

And you don't deserve to be either. Should this ever happen, if you don't feel confident speaking to the PT directly, please tell the reception or management, vote with your money and leave them.

Fitter Confident You Client Stories: Joe Luebke

I was very active in my 20s and 30s. I played competitive volleyball and had a physically demanding job - I was in good shape. My lifestyle became more sedentary in my 40s and I started to put on the pounds. I started working out at the work gym but didn't really know what I was doing. I'd do cardio for an hour and lift some weights on the machines but steered clear of free weights. I certainly didn't want anyone to think I didn't know what I was doing on the free weights! I started doing organized classes in the gym and loved them.

Even though I ate well, I ate too much. Bottom line was, even though I was working out, I wasn't seeing much progress.

I joined the Fitter Confident Youniverse in January 2020. The first programme I did with Matt was the LEAN group. I thoroughly enjoyed the programme and group of men and it was successful beyond my imagination. I've made friends with people I would never have met. Everyone in the group wants you to succeed and with Matt's guidance and cheerleading, you can succeed. Everything came together in a holistic manner that I'd never really been able to crack before. Nutrition, workouts, mental health: it all clicked. I ended up taking off nearly 30 pounds in that first programme.

I've continued working with Matt on solo programmes and group programmes. Being nearly 60 years old, I'm the strongest and healthiest I've been since my 20s. Working with Matt was a life-changing decision and I know I can continue to take care of my body and age gracefully and with strength.

AGE, AGING & AGEISM

WITHIN OUR COMMUNITY, ESPECIALLY WITH GAY males, there has long been an obsession with youth and staying young - the male Beauty Industry in the UK is worth more than £500 million a year (Sumup Business Guide https://bit.ly/3yTvi3m) and growing. Ditto the world of Botox, fillers and online filters.

How that plays out in my world is speaking with people who feel they've left it too late. They might **say** they think it's too late to get fit, strong and build their confidence, but underneath, there's usually an element of:

 'Too late to get the body I want, that I've been trained to believe will make me happy and unlock untold confidence and contentment."

SOME IMPORTANT POINTS:

1. There are people with 'that' body who are deeply unhappy
2. There are people who've never done a day of exercise in their life, who have absolutely unbridled happiness and will never not feel fabulous
3. Your version of 'that body' is actually different to everyone else's interpretation
4. Holding this belief is deferring and holding off you being happy right here, right now. It's the same as 'I'll be happy when I lose X kg' – No, you won't. It's not about the number on the scales
5. And the most important one of all: you have not left it too late - whatever 'it' is.

I'm grateful to be working with some clients in their 60s who are the fittest, strongest and most proud of themselves they've ever been - and I have no doubt Fitter Confident You could support and improve the lives of people in their 70s and older.

But why this drive for some mysterious, ageless 'perfection'?

Social media's grasp on our collective consciousness of course plays a part, and not just in LGBTQ+ people.

But that aside, here's why I believe so many of us cling to the vestiges of youth:

Firstly, many of us - certainly those born in the last century (!) - just didn't have the adolescence, teenage years, 20s and even

30s or later that we really wanted, as we couldn't be our true selves.

Having to hide my sexuality at home, at school, even with friends, created a facade I hid behind; an alternate persona who - of course! - fancied girls and definitely didn't just hang around with them because he preferred their company.

Society then just felt like it didn't allow this - everyone was straight, that was the rule, and that was how we all had to play it.

Watching *Heartstopper* on Netflix recently was a joy - the acceptance! The normalisation! The curtains! (both fabric and follicle)... but as mentioned it was a million miles removed from my school experience in the 80s and 90s.

So, when you can't have those important years the way you would have liked them to be at the time, when you grow up and gain financial and social independence, opportunities start to present to allow you to relive your lost years - and yes, clawing back some essence of youth can be part of that.

Then the link to our focus on aging and attaining some mythically 'perfect' body is twofold:

1. Present as straight as possible

"Well I'm gay but I'm not *that* gay" - if you're attracted to men in some way, you're gay or bi or queer, there are no semantics to be argued over here.

No one is forcing you to come out in any part of your life. Yes, sexuality as a whole is a spectrum, but the notion that because you wear suits and watch Match of the Day, you're less gay than someone in a (fabulous) pink crop top doesn't stand up and is just a projection of internalised homophobia.

Acceptance of our own self, life, character and dreams is the best way out of this - after all, if you can't accept yourself, how in the hell are you going to accept someone else?

This links to the concept of 'Passing Privilege'; two men walking down a street in 'traditional' clothes usually won't be noticed. They have the 'privilege' to 'pass' as straight, so get to carry on with their days without any further scrutiny.

But those who are brave enough to wear what they want, when they want; who hold hands or kiss in crowded places, risking - unbelievably in 2022 - homophobic attacks, they are the ones who make bold steps forward for all of us.

It blows my mind that holding your partner's hand in public is still a political act, but when the rights of my community are being challenged and rescinded all over the world, it is.

This isn't some defiant rallying cry - your safety and wellbeing is paramount.

It's also not my intention to paint the world outside your front door as unforgiving and dangerous. Plus we all have our own personal battles, struggles and to-do lists each day, so please don't feel it's your responsibility to solve all these problems, it's not.

But if the time is right, know that you being your amazing, true self will always be a lighthouse for someone else in the dark. You may not even know whose pathway you've suddenly lit up, but our visibility, honesty and truthfulness is one of the best ways we grow as a community.

2. Present as healthy as possible

THIS IS HEAVIER STILL: I'll be discussing HIV and AIDS.

Covid-19 isn't the only global pandemic of our times, yet it's frequently discussed as if it is.

It's absolutely not a competition about who has it worst, but AIDS has killed more than 6 times as many people as Covid - 6.2 million from Covid, 36.6 million from HIV and AIDS. (World Health Organisation: https://bit.ly/3AGk2bL)

I was born in 1981, so only have the vaguest of real memories of the crisis at its worst - a photo in a magazine of a man wasting away in a hospital bed; playground insults (to anyone, not me specifically), but as far removed as I was, it still felt like a menacing spectre, hanging over all of us.

SIDE NOTE:

I've already mentioned the damage done by the Conservative Party policies of the time that forbade the 'promotion' of homosexuality in school; the information I received about it was always second-, third-, fourth-hand and of course twisted and incorrect.

I'd love to say we've moved on and those in charge have realised that when you try to ban or hide things there are only negative repercussions... But we haven't. It's literally happening again, right now, in Florida, with the 'Don't say gay' Bill passed earlier this year, again, forbidding the discussion in schools of any relationship other than the hetero-normative.

The right wing lobby behind this seem to believe that the LGBTQ+ agenda is to teach primary school children about gay sex. In reality, any reasonable person would realise it's just to allow teachers to explain that some children have a Mummy and Daddy, some have two Mummies, some have two Daddies, some just have one parent etc. etc. etc. until my head falls off.

It's the same with the potential move to ban abortions in America. This won't stop people having abortions, it will only force people to have unsafe abortions.

I need to stop this side note before I get so angry I can't type any more.

WITH THE AIDS CRISIS, and the media and government's output that it was predominantly a disease gay men caught, came three things:

1. That being gay was dangerous and made you an outlier
2. That you were going to get AIDS and die
3. That to be accepted you had to prove you were fit and healthy and strong and therefore less likely to be gay.

There's a twisted logic to using your body and its muscle as the reason behind your actions:

- The more muscle I have, the more 'masculine' I look
- The more 'masculine' I look, the more like 'a man' I look
- Therefore, I can pass for straight and be accepted by the world and not get AIDS
- Therefore, the more muscle I have, the straighter I can be, the safer I will be.

This didn't exist in its own silo - bodybuilding and fitness had been growing in popularity since the 70s - now working out and improving your personal fitness was easier than ever.

Which leads me to steroids.

All - ALL - of the famous competitive bodybuilders from the 70s on - yes, Arnold too - took steroids to speed up and enhance the muscle-building process.

This was never about strength or fitness, it was purely about size and muscle form and winning bodybuilding competitions.

I've just been researching steroid use (or PEDs as they're more commonly called now - performance enhancing drugs) and almost fell off my chair on discovering - from multiple sources - that in the UK alone in 2019, up to 1 million people were using them.

One million people.

One million people, most of whom won't understand the intricacies of their use, risking their health for the assumed goal of growing a bigger body. Because...?

It opens doors? So they can be an influencer online? Get invited to parties? They'll be happier? Sleep with as many people as possible / find the perfect partner? All of the above?

Actually, none of the above. Not really.

All of this speaks to the need for external validation - getting the approval of others or society in general.

I know that can be alluring - I used to post topless shots online with the hope for as many likes as possible - but it's ultimately hollow and isn't a sustainable path to happiness.

Doing what you love, what lights you up, being in the flow with those elements, is what brings happiness as it isn't actually a destination.

That's where the people thinking that losing X kilos will make them happy are going wrong - seeing happiness as a destination at which you can arrive, when it's really finding the joy in what you do, that brings happiness into your life - and then keeps you doing those things. It really is a journey, one which you have the power to define and manoeuvre where and how you like.

All of this is to say you deserve every happiness.

Changing your body for someone else's reasons is not how you achieve that.

Doing good things for yourself and the world around you, inspiring those who need it (when you can), brings the motivation back in to you, your dreams and your reasons why.

If you want to, please do build a strong, healthy, resilient mind and body - a wonderful process and gift for yourself and the world - but do it for you, for how it makes you feel, for the confidence and self-belief it gives you to go out there and be the best, happiest, most grounded version of you that you can be.

INTERLUDE
CHECK-IN WITH GEORGE

YOU MAY REMEMBER FROM THE INTRODUCTION, WE met a man called George, who had had some good intentions and the motivation to do something positive for himself.

He threw himself into getting up early and hitting the treadmill; he cut out all the 'bad' food he had been eating and decided 'this was it', he was going to be healthy for good.

Unfortunately, that's not how it worked out.

Everything George chose to do was just too full-on, too extreme, too different to what he'd been doing before, so the gym membership went to waste, the guilt and shame returned and he felt, more than ever, that fitness was what other people did.

He did, at least, decide to cancel his gym membership.

A few months passed. Work was busy, quieter, busy, quieter; George went for the odd jog but nothing really changed... Until someone new joined his team at work.

He guessed Alessandro was a similar age, but didn't look as tired as George did. Over the first few weeks, George found out he was gay, had a partner and was in fact, the exact same age. He seemed to eat pretty much what other people did and he had joined the team for after work drinks a couple of times too.

So, George started trying to discover what his secret was, what revolutionary tips he was utilising that gave him energy and confidence...

Which turned out not to be revolutionary or 'hacks' of any kind at all... Which at first was annoying, as it meant there was no shortcut to where George wanted to be...

But then it was reassuring as it meant he hadn't been kept out of some great secret that everyone knew apart from him!

Over time, with the guidance of a friend (who was a PT), Alessandro had started to implement a few things which didn't seem like much, but they'd been easy to stick to, so he'd stuck to them and it turned out they were contributing to him feel a bit fitter and a bit more confident too.

He had started to drink a bit more water - he still had one or two cans of Diet Coke a day, but had previously been drinking four or more, so, very steadily, weaned himself off them.

He started lifting weights for 20 minutes, three times a week. He did this at home for six months and then moved to a local gym.

"No cardio?" said George.

"No," said Alessandro.

George was gob smacked.

Alessandro had also started eating a bit more protein and-

"Oh, I don't want to be a gym bunny, chugging protein shakes." said George.

"You don't have to use them. I just find one for breakfast convenient," said Alessandro.

And that was basically it.

Over time, he'd started to try other things - a class at this gym, meditating now and then, a bit of yoga - but none of it required anything too extreme or a drastic overhaul of his life and it was all because he wanted to try these things. There was no pressure for him to do anything other than that which would help him feel good or stronger, just... better.

"So, no dieting?" asked George.

"No. I had dieted before, but the diets didn't teach me anything other than how to do that diet. So, when I stopped the diet, I didn't know how to eat in the real world again. Since then, I've started learning a bit about how food works, what's in what I'm eating, and that was enough to help me make slightly different choices about what to eat. Or just reduce my portion sizes a bit."

This was news to George and the opposite of everything he'd tried before. It sort-of sounded too good to be true, but it wasn't like he'd had any success doing anything like this in the past.

George went home with lots to think about.

Fitter Confident You Client Stories: Mark Pattison

When I turned 40, I promised myself to make my health and wellbeing a priority, particularly spurred on by a health scare in my 20s. Over the next couple of years, I tried a handful of fitness programmes, some with an unsustainable 'balls to the wall' attitude, and most with limited success.

I came across Fitter Confident You during lockdown, at a point where I was feeling quite frustrated and cynical about fitness because it just hadn't clicked with me. I'd severely pulled my back out on a previous programme - I literally felt broken - and having consumed various fitness myths, believed that my body was incapable of coping with heavy weights and that reaching any ideal level of fitness was a pipe dream.

But… I stuck to the first Fitter Confident You workouts and kept reminding myself of the genuine testimonials from guys like myself, who all reassured me that significant transformation was achievable. By the end of the first four weeks I remember doing a double take in a mirror, suddenly noticing how quickly my belly had shrunk.

That first surprise was a satisfying moment, and it's those unexpected changes that have been most rewarding and have given me newfound confidence that a dream level of fitness is completely within reach, given time, patience, and faith that the basics are all that you need to make a difference.

I love that fitness is now just a natural part of my lifestyle; it doesn't feel like a chore, or a struggle to fit in. And, dare I say it, I enjoy it! I haven't had to make huge changes either, just incremental tweaks here and there.

When I joined Fitter Confident You, I didn't believe that my sexuality played any part in my health and fitness mindset; I have never knowingly experienced homophobia, but quickly came to realise just how much I'd unconsciously held myself back in straighter fitness environments, whether that was feeling intimidated by groups of straight lads hogging the weights at the gym, or asking for help and feeling dismissed by PTs who seemed more focused on impressing their female client base.

Learning to let my guard down and be myself within the Fitter Confident You community has proved fundamental in changing my mindset and approach to fitness.

Improving physical health is one thing, but I feel more mentally comfortable in my own skin and it's amazing how taking full control of your overall wellbeing in that way is like pouring a truck-load of cement into the foundations of what makes you tick as a human being, which is a wonderfully calming and peaceful place to be.

BIG MO (AND HOW TO FIND IT!)

"HOW CAN I GET MOTIVATED?" AND "HOW CAN I FIND motivation?" are the two questions I get asked the most.

After that, it's "how can I build fitness/strength/confidence?" but the thing is, if you haven't got motivation to take any steps forward, then your fitness/strength/confidence is unlikely to change.

So, let's start with motivation. Specifically, let's look at why you're not feeling motivated to move.

Physical Reasons

Is work particularly busy? Are you going through anything stressful in your personal life? When we have to use extra mental bandwidth dealing with events out of the ordinary, it can zap our drive to do other things, as much as we know they might be of benefit.

Linked to this, you might still be thinking you need to find an hour at a time to get any benefits, but that's not the case. Even just 10-15 minutes a few times a week can start to make a big difference, in two ways:

- How you feel there and then - a flush of positive hormones (endorphins) to lift you up
- How you feel long term - these feelings of accomplishment and action are great for your self-esteem and self-belief, not to mention overall stress reduction, improved likelihood of better sleep, better mood and energy levels the next day, and so on and so on.

Also, are you surrounded by naysayers? These could be at home, the office, online or anywhere you hang out.

If you predominantly spend your time with people who don't exercise and don't see the point of starting, then you're already on the back foot, as - trust me - there are a billion people out there who DO and would love to cheer you on.

Another physical reason is to do with convenience.

The most important factor to consider when choosing a gym is the location. It HAS to be convenient to either home or work, otherwise you're unlikely to stick at it. A 30-minute walk or commute will seem more and more off-putting and on any days with Low Mo, it will most likely be another hurdle in the way of getting you moving.

If there isn't a gym nearby, start with home workouts - a pair of dumbbells that you can roll under the bed in the spare room is all you need - meaning within five minutes of finishing work, you can be working out.

Emotional Reasons

There's a lot to be said for knowing why you're doing something, and even more so if that 'why' has a powerful emotional attachment.

I'd always encourage your reasons to be your own, not from society or peer-pressure. BUT, if those sorts of motivations are what it takes to get you moving, then use them to get started, but adjust and improve them as you get into your rhythm.

For example, if you have a holiday in the diary and believe you need to lose X kg to enjoy it, then yes, start with that. I can promise you that when you get to that weight, you'll see that it hasn't actually changed anything but like I said, if that's what it takes to get you into a routine, I'll take it for now.

What I'd then suggest is starting to get in touch with all the other wonderful things that are happening, all the myriad ways you're progressing and feeling better, and focusing on getting more of them.

Which is another handy point: are you focusing on what you've got to lose (or what you will lose)? For example:

- I have to lose weight
- I have to change who I am
- I'll have to cut out all my favourite foods so will miss out on eating out, dinner parties

- I'll lose time (with my friends, doing my favourite things etc.)

Look how miserable all those reasons sound.

Of course you wouldn't stick to a plan if those were the thoughts underneath it all. I wouldn't!

Going into it, you would see it all like a chore, like something you have to force yourself to do, then, unsurprisingly, it would *feel* like a chore and why on earth would you consciously make time for anything that felt like a chore?

The kinder, much more sustainable and enjoyable way to approach getting into the ol' fitness is to look at what you have to GAIN. Let's go over some of those reasons again, as they bear repeating:

- Strength!
- Mental resilience!
- Self-belief!
- Speed!
- Sleep!
- Energy!
- Mood!
- Sex drive!
- Confidence!
- New friends!
- New skills!
- Better balance and coordination!

- Greater bone density! (admittedly, not very sexy BUT should you fall over, you'll be less likely to break a bone, so actually, quite useful, no?!)
- And yes, TIME - when you have more energy, you're in a better mood more often, get ill *less* often, you actually have more time and drive to do the things you love, with the people you love.

Fitter Confident Client Stories: Darren Chadwick-Hussein

What was my life like back then? It now feels like One Million Years B(F)C(Y). I neglected my health and wellbeing, life was pretty much like every Lana Del Ray song. The only time I did an ab crunch was when I sat up in bed to light a cigarette. I'd perfected the Subtle Art of Not Giving A F*ck way before it became a New York Times Bestseller. Was I happy? In a way. Was something missing? Very much so.

After getting married I did the typical thing of ballooning in weight. Going from nine stone to fourteen really takes a lot of commitment. And Jacob's Creek. So I sobered up and joined a gym.

It was a very gay gym. Very. VERY. The sort of place where if you sat on the changing room bench for too long you'd catch an STI.

It didn't bother me, I wasn't a practising homosexual; I didn't need to practice, I was already very good at it. But I found it too intimidating: there's talk of 'gay currency' - where your worth is tied to your age and your appearance. And I was more Car Boot Sale than Wall Street. Gay Currency equals Money and Money talks. Money for me said 'there are insufficient funds in your account'.

What felt like years of working out with minimal progress was having a negative effect on me. I was five minutes away from giving Mephistopheles a holler to make a deal when I scrolled through Facebook and an ad appeared.

Fitter You Global.

And its creator: Matt Boyles. Perfect hair, perfect teeth, perfect lean physique. I immediately hated every fibre of his being.

But I was always taught not to judge people on appearances, so I thought I'd investigate further to give me better reasons to hate him.

He seemed friendly. He wasn't like other trainers I'd seen online. The more I dug the harder it was to resist. After being impressed with his rapport and energy I made a decision: Matt's the only online personal trainer I wouldn't request a urine sample from before handing over my money.

And so it began.

In storytelling your main character has a want but actually has a more important need.

And Matt had a great way of cutting through that, as the truth was, above any body goal, what I really needed was to reclaim my self-belief that had been buried long ago.

Physical exercise and mental well-being should go hand in hand but often one is neglected for the sake of the other. Sure, that guy in the magazine may have a sixpack you could grate cheese on but have you thought about the internal battles and insecurities he may be fighting?

Matt set tasks. They weren't the Labours of Hercules but certainly challenged me (in a good way). No spoilers - do the course yourself and they are peppered throughout this book - but they got to the heart of the matter.

And he revealed secrets. The reason I was still skinny? Diet. I needed carbs more than anything.

My new BFF. They gave me the clay to make the pot. Before I hadn't enough clay to even make an ashtray. He also revealed He Man was actually Prince Adam but that's a story for another time.

I'd become fitter and I'd become more confident. I'd achieved my 'need'. I didn't care what anyone else thought. I cared about me. You should try it, it's very liberating.

Thank you Matt for opening the door.

HOW TO BUILD YOUR GYMFIDENCE

Gymfidence – Noun: confidence in the gym or while working out.

You've decided you want to get fit and start a bit of the ol' fitness – good for you!

Exercise environments (and even just the concept of exercise) can sometimes seem intimidating, but this is usually just our perception of them, aka, the unknown = scary.

However, getting comfortable so you can just quietly get on with your workout doesn't take as long as you may think. You will have experienced this in other areas of your life, but remember this phrase: with competence, comes confidence! So, to speed up the process, here are 10 handy tips to get you started:

1. Figure out when your gym is quietest and go then - if
    you Google the specific branch of your gym, it will tell
    you this – which is handy!
2. Go with a friend - sounds obvious, but if you've never
    tried it, it will transform the experience. You get
    accountability, someone to push you, someone to spot
    you, someone to halve any embarrassment you might
    feel; it's fun!
3. Put your headphones on AND your phone on flight
    mode. Spotify & Audible let you download
    songs/books so you can go in and be undisturbed by
    the outside world - letting exercise become your
    meditation. Your favourite songs and podcast can help
    you power through and stay focused on what you're
    there to do.
4. Have a plan and practise it beforehand. With
    competence comes confidence - if you know what
    you're doing, you can just walk in there and do what
    you want to do. Watch videos in advance, even
    practise the moves at home or at a free gym in the
    park, and after a few times you'll be a pro…
5. Or just do home workouts. They can be just as
    effective as a gym workout and it removes any
    external stresses. Buy a 5kg pair of dumbbells if you're
    just starting out, and take it from there.
6. Or in fact, do you want/need to be there? If you've
    tried the gym before and just don't get on with it,
    that's A-OK. There are hundreds of different ways to
    build health and fitness into your life, you don't have
    to go to a gym if it's not your thing.

7. Treat yourself to some new workout clothes and trainers - it's modern armour and can inspire you to step it up. Plus, it doesn't have to break the bank; TK Maxx always has a great sportswear section and the Christmas sales always have bargains!

8. Work with a professional to learn from the best; all gyms should offer you at least one free session to get started and the PTs in your gym may give you a session too, as they want your business - don't be afraid to ask and try a few out to see who suits you and your goals.

9. Take a step back and ask yourself WHY you're there. Just to get fitter is fine, but maybe you've got a child and want to be able to carry her without getting out of breath, or maybe you want to build confidence to apply for a new job - finding a deeper motivation can be amazing.

10. Think about how much money you're wasting every time you don't go - the more you go, the cheaper it becomes pro rata. Two sessions a month at £30 a visit, just to use the treadmill may not be the best use of your funds...

So there you go!

And there will be more - your own ones, for example! I love hearing new ways to help people get started, so if you'd like to add something, email me on matt@fitteryou.net, and I'll share them on my social media channels!

Fitter Confident You Client Stories: Matthew Bridle (and
Nigel Boarer)

Despite having had a life-long desire to be thinner, fitter and
quite frankly, more attractive, life never seemed to allow for
much personal development. Never having been a sporty
chap, either at school or subsequently, coupled with being a
bit of a foodie and coming from a long line of chunky males,
my physical state was never something that I could be
proud of.

Getting undressed in front of anyone else, or the prospect of a
day at the beach, filled me with utter trepidation. Over the
years, I had made several attempts at dieting, some successful,
others torturously pointless. As middle age advanced, I was
aware that my waistline was also developing whilst my
general fitness levels were decreasing, and so, in late 2019, I
began looking around on the internet for trainers and
programmes.... but just looking and without much (or any)
commitment.

I stumbled across Matt and Fitter Confident You and thought
'perhaps, after Christmas it might be something to do'.
Christmas came and went and I did nothing about it.

In February 2020, I was away working in Switzerland when
the Pandemic really took hold: within a couple of weeks, all
my work for the year had been cancelled and I returned home.

The first week of the Pandemic was brilliant... Lunchtime
drinking, box sets on the telly: our house was two-man party-
central for a week - no colleagues, fancy meals and lots of
booze. After a week of literally rolling around on the sofa, I

had a mail drop from Matt; The latest L E A N programme was about to start, there were spaces left. In one split second, my life changed. Seriously, I'm not even being overly dramatic.

I signed up and began almost immediately. I had reached a point where, in all honesty, I found my own body repugnant and I needed help. The L E A N programme, coupled with Matt's live daily midday workout, gave me a structure, a goal and a purpose. The feeling of being part of a supportive community, being part of a tribe, the jokes, the banter, the support from both Matt and the community, just ignited something within me which totally changed my outlook on everything.

The L E A N programme was an education for me: I was totally ignorant as to what a calorie deficit was. I learnt that nothing had to be a trial or a burden, no food was off-limits and that the combination of sticking to a calorie limit per day combined with easy regular physical exercise was the key to success.

Not two weeks had passed of religiously following the plan when the changes to my body and to my outlook began to change: my husband, who initially expressed no interest or desire to join me on a personal development journey, became curious.

He started eating the same things as me, reducing portion sizes and limiting alcohol intake. Before long, we were both following the plan, and without the influences of the outside world during lockdown, both our shapes and fitness began to change dramatically.

Matt had ignited in us both, not only with the desire to invest time and energy in ourselves but also by showing us that through steady, regular exercise, even in our 50s there was still potential to be realised; that age is just a number and that anything is possible. At the end of the summer, we both signed up to do a twelve-week programme with Matt: for us, it was the perfect balance of flexibility and support, totally adaptable to circumstance.

We both just kept on becoming fitter, leaner and indeed, more confident. We began achieving physical goals which had seemed impossibly unobtainable prior to working with Matt. The first weights were purchased, then replaced with heavier ones and new clothes had to be bought. The 36" jeans which I used to squeeze into were superseded by 31". As life began to return to normality, travel and work began to recommence, with all the distractions that came with it too. We continued doing what we had learnt with Matt.

Four twelve-week programmes later, with several phases of, let's say, reduced involvement, the foundations and knowledge are a consistent part of our lives. Yes, we go on holiday and throw caution to the wind, eat and drink far too much, but the education and training that we received serve as a constant guide and a reminder of what we need to do. We are different people now: we do our best to schedule our exercise into our daily lives. We make choices which some of our friends find inexplicable and rather unnecessary. We take a set of weights and a couple of mats with us when we go away in the car - when we fly, we take our trainers for running.

I would never have believed that the fat, asthmatic kid would have become so addicted to exercise and a physical, healthy lifestyle. The point is, however, that we both feel FANTAS-TIC, energised and confident.

I am calmer, less stressed, less easily annoyed or wound up by others, kinder to myself, less critical. I love my new shape, it's by no means perfect, but a successful work in progress.

We have made good friends, tried new things, accepted new challenges and have never been fitter or healthier in the almost three decades that we have been together. We are currently revising our latest 12-week plan using Matt's brilliant workout app, before signing up for another 12 weeks in the autumn.

Fitter Confident You and the utterly brilliant, charming, funny and charismatic Matt have changed our lives and I couldn't be happier or more grateful.

WHY THIS WON'T WORK FOR YOU

THERE'S JUST ONE REASON WHY THIS WON'T WORK for you.

But first off, here's another (non-exhaustive) list of things that have NO bearing on whether or not you can get into a routine with your fitness and wellbeing:

- Your job
- The hours you work
- Your height
- Your weight
- You age
- Your genetics
- Your income
- Your sleeping patterns
- Your chosen way of eating - i.e., vegan or omnivore
- Your previous experience

- Your preferred location for working out - i.e., gym, home, park
- Your workout gear
- Your trainers
- Your Internet connection!

The only thing that will stop this working for you, is your willingness to give it a chance.

Whatever your previous experience or beliefs around your fitness and wellbeing, the Fitter Confident You approach of baby steps, empathy, kindness, breathing space, and humour means this works. And I know it works as it's worked for more than 1,000 people, just like you, all around the world.

I know some of you have had negative experiences with fitness and the Fitness Industry. I've heard some horror stories of PTs shaming their clients:

"I can't believe you didn't go for a run this weekend"

"If you're not tracking every calorie you may as well not track any of them"

"This was years ago, but I had a trainer who kept making judgmental comments about other people in the gym, but quietly so they wouldn't hear. Apart from it being just rude, I kept having to remind him to focus on me. Also, he was really only quasi-encouraging: he was basically supportive during our sessions but just the opposite when it came to what I wanted to do with fitness. Me: "I'd like to train for a 10k this fall." Him: "Yeah there's no way you'll be ready by then. Not even close." Thanks, you jerk."

"Turned up to a PT session, a guy I'd been seeing for four months and was paying £80 an hour, full of a cold but I didn't want to cancel on him, and he said he didn't think I was trying hard enough and that I was wasting his time. Safe to say it was my last session with him. Also during the time I was seeing him he seemed more concerned about how we could market my progress on his social media, rather than the progress I was actually looking to make, so in that regard, I probably was wasting his time!"

"A number of years ago now but a PT had me do an incline chest press that was too heavy and I tore several muscles that had me out for months."

"A trainer insisted I had to eat meat if I wanted to make gains and, since he was the professional and I was paying for it, I did it for six months until I ended our contract." [This from a vegan!]

"How about the trainer who was hell-bent on making me vomit and feel useless by lots of medicine ball slams followed by an incline TRX row, virtually horizontal to the ground - despite me saying I hadn't trained for 5 years and just wanted to do basics to get going again. Basically set me an impossible routine to boost his own ego and deflate mine."

"When I was learning to swim I was most definitely the slowest swimmer in the group. To speed me up, the trainer got a brush, a proper yard brush for sweeping, and every time I dropped below the desired speed, he would whack me with the brush. Needless to say I hated it and it did nothing for my skin either!"

"I was told: 'You really should just push through your illness and compete in the CrossFit open... sweating will make you feel better...' (I had pneumonia and a fever of 104)"

These are genuine quotes from members of the free Fitter Confident You group.

There are also those unpleasant situations where the client has asked for a break or to ease off a bit, and the PT has forced them to push ahead. At best, this leaves the client with a bad taste in their mouth about the experience; at worst, this leads to injury.

The thing is, it's just so easy to not do it like this.

To listen.

To pause.

To understand that everyone works at different speeds and intensities AND that everyone's experience is relative only to their unique way of perceiving the world around them - that is, one man's 50% effort is another's all out.

The other piece of the puzzle is to listen to yourself too.

This was something I ignored - at my own cost - for far too long.

I used to have such a 'push-through-at-all-costs' mentality, and really hurt myself twice because of it. So, to be clear, if you're doing any exercise, any move, in any class, and you feel anything out of the ordinary, STOP!

It may well be you just need to pause and have a stretch, or click your elbow or knee and all is lined up and working how it should be again... OR it could be a warning sign in the form of a light or mild strain, that could very easily be exacerbated.

Much better to finish a workout early and be able to go back in a day or two, than foolishly try to push through, *really* hurt yourself and then be out of action for two weeks.

I learned this the hard way with both squats and deadlifts, but now will always stop and reassess what's going on, and finish a session if necessary.

None of this is to scare you; it's to take off any pressure you might ever feel from your workouts. As you progress, you will naturally lift heavier weights, and the more that happens, the more you have to be in tune with your body, but please don't let this put you off.

And I now squat and deadlift safely and happily!

Figuring out a workout routine that lifts me up on a daily basis has been one of the biggest joys of my life. It has absolutely transformed who I am, what I do and how I show up in the world, and it can absolutely be all that for you too.

Fitter Confident You Client Stories: Jack Coleman

Before I joined the Fitter Confident Youniverse, I had been doing my own workouts based upon my previous experience. I was doing okay. Well enough. But I felt I could/should be doing better. I knew that it was a nutrition issue. I considered going back to the nutritionist I worked with in 2020 who helped me shed my 30 pounds of COVID lockdown fat (I lost 40, regained 10). I decided to do FCY instead because I felt certain Matt would give challenging workouts as well as sound nutrition guidance. True on both accounts!

As of this writing, I have one official week left of the program. I have more lean muscle and am very pleased. I intend to cycle through the twelve weeks again, increasing weights where safely appropriate; but it was also suggested I might do a week of each phase in order, which sounds like a great idea.

I learned that, even though I already have a solid knowledge base on how to create effective workouts, I kept doing the same things, which slowed my progress. It's very helpful to get input from someone else. They will likely be more challenging and maybe even remind you of exercises you forgot about. I'm so happy I did it!

BEATING THE FITNESS INDUSTRY AT ITS OWN GAME

AKA, THE PROBLEM WITH THE FITNESS INDUSTRY.

If you don't see yourself represented in something, then why would you feel welcomed or encouraged to join it?

Part of the problem me and my clients have faced, is not feeling welcomed in the Fitness Industry.

There's been a huge shift in the last 10 years, to a more inclusive approach, partly due to the explosion in numbers of jobs available in gyms, leisure centres, hotel fitness centres and from the sheer volume of people becoming Personal Trainers.

But rewind just a bit further back and fitness wasn't seen as a particularly glamorous or dynamic profession – it was a fall back option for people (mainly boys) who didn't do that well at school. So it's not hard to see why a similar, unwelcoming atmosphere pervaded gyms: the PTs who went on work in gyms were the same people who made PE miserable for so many.

The power the memories those formative school experiences can still wield over us can't be underestimated – many FCY clients have discussed how they always felt singled out by PE teachers, some even being insulted and called names. So, it stands to reason why people feel uncomfortable in gym environments; the changing rooms, the loud, seemingly hypermasculine 'free weights' area, the fear of standing out for the wrong reasons, the range of new equipment to master... Not to mention feeling physically exposed too. We sometimes underestimate how clothes we feel comfortable in allow us to get on with our days more easily, but someone changed into a pair of shorts and t-shirt can feel even more vulnerable in a new environment, which is only exacerbated by the pressure of having to show off their physical prowess *and* being reminded of unpleasant school memories.

I've had my share of these experiences.

Walking into a gym, feeling uncomfortable, getting on the treadmill and going home after 15 minutes.

And *then* we have to add in the stress of having to come out... More on that later!

Plus - oh God, when will it stop?! - not to mention how the Fitness Industry has typically always presented itself.

Of COURSE some part of what we do is about aspiration. Showing what's possible. Demonstrating how good it can feel.

How that was usually translated was with pictures of gym-honed bodies, positioned as the pinnacle of physical wellbeing. If there were faces, they were moody and serious, meaning you must take fitness seriously, fitness is a serious business and you better bloody take your fitness seriously if you're going to do it properly. And the images were in black and white of course, because colour photos would be too frivolous and not serious enough.

Yawn.

So, let's summarise how the Fitness Industry has chosen to present itself over the years:

- Hard
- Serious
- For tough people
- Unwelcoming
- Very much a boy's club
- A serious endeavour
- Unfun (that's a word)
- Did I mention serious?

No wonder it was so stagnant for so long and I have welcomed with open arms the way it has finally – *finally!* – started to evolve.

The democratisation of fitness, meaning more and more good value, accessible gyms with more and more advertising, encouraging everybody – and every body – that finding their own rhythm with their wellbeing is possible, is a very good thing.

Right at the start of when I created Fitter Confident You, I knew instinctively how I wanted the company to work and why it was different.

It would be fun. There would be jokes and humour. There would be bags of empathy. There would be the most inclusive and supportive community people had ever been part of. I wanted to be the anti-Fitness Industry; to prove it could be done a very different way, and still get great results. Better, in fact.

I didn't have a manifesto, but I've since written one, to which I regularly refer, to ensure everything FCY is and does sticks to it as closely as possible:

1. Everyone must feel welcome and included – that this IS something they can do and it IS something they will want to keep going
2. When faced with the options to be right or to be kind, choose kindness, always
3. Everything must be easy to understand and jargon-free - meaning someone on their very first day of putting on trainers will understand what to do, how to do it, and WHY they're doing it
4. I will never talk about appearance in my content or advertising; yes, your physical appearance will change when you get into a routine with your workouts and nutrition, but I always encourage clients to move that down their list of priorities
5. I will inspire and encourage clients to look and learn to appreciate the widest range of possible metrics, from more energy, to higher sex drive, better sleep, to exploding strength, better mood, faster runs, and clearer skin

6. I will lead from the front and lead by example, with humour and good will.

Fitter Confident You Client Stories: Ian Dawe

Why did I start (and continue!) to workout? To future proof myself against the wear and tear of life's pressures, both mentally and physically, now and as I grow older; to feel fitter, stronger, to sleep better and to really do something good for me, long term.

Seeing the results of the work I put in is such a driver for me - it's almost three years since we first started working together - how did that happen?! *I'd love to be able to meet my former self and tell them what good things were around the corner.*

I enjoy the workouts and do them on my terms - baby steps, as Matt says - it really is all about habit and with the FCY guidance and support, seeing and feeling the changes in my body and the confidence that comes with that.

Over the last three years I've some important lessons:

- How to destroy/break the cycle of food/exercise reward/sin
- Understanding that it matters not one bit if I miss a workout or something gets in the way; reassess; restart
- Instead of avoiding working out due to tiredness, or taking the easy way out, realising that exercise actually makes me feel so much better - i.e., feeling the release of those happy hormones
- Learning and accepting my own limitations, and the difference between challenging myself and pushing myself too far

- We are all different shapes and sizes. Social Media is the worst place to seek comfort - approval comes from within, not Instagram and Twitter.

I love where I've got to and am excited to keep going - onwards!

COURAGE, BRAVERY & DOING THE RIGHT THING

THE VERY ACT OF STEPPING OUTSIDE OUR HOUSES...
The very act of our *existence* as LGBTQ+ people is political.

I'd rather it wasn't, but when our validity is put to a vote to an entire country, and subject to 'banter' on social media on a minute-by-minute basis, being LGBTQ+ is absolutely political.

This doesn't mean you have to go to demonstrations, or write to your MP on the daily and in an ideal world, it wouldn't be on us to educate and change the system, as it wouldn't need changing... But it does. A lot.

However, I also appreciate that we're busy enough as it is, and our own personal lives are just as important - our own struggles, wins, relationships, ups, down, sideways movements - so when we ladle in 'bringing about fundamental systemic change', it's no wonder it can all feel a bit much, and life in general can feel tiring.

Consider National Coming Out Day (Tuesday 11th October in 2022 - mark your filo-faxes!) a lovely idea to remind the world that Coming Out is still a thing we have to do.

Should you not be LGBTQ+, you would be forgiven for assuming it was a 'once-and-done' scenario. You've come out to your family and friends - great! Now let's get the bus to G.A.Y. and dance to Holly Valance's second album (*Desire* - I know you knew that) for a few hours.

Wrong!

Every day, sometimes multiple times a day, we have to come out.

Meet someone new and talk for long enough and you'll invariably get to discussions about partners, relationships etc.

And it's tiring, and even in the most apparently liberal and safest of areas, there's always a chance of the conversation turning sour, or worse.

This is unless you hide it and obfuscate the truth - and I don't blame you if you choose that route. One time in Sainsbury's a woman asked me how the kids were, and I just said "oh, they're fine..." and prayed she didn't dig any deeper. This was really more of a case of mistaken identity, but in the split-second of deciding what answer to give, I was still confronted with the option to out myself to a complete stranger by the tills and those around me, not knowing precisely what the outcome would be.

This takes courage and resilience, and for a myriad of reasons, our resilience levels go up and down, catch us in a lower ebb and I may still take the path of least resistance... which is so sad.

However, it's through brave people leaning into those uncomfortable moments that breakthroughs and progress are made... And I ducked out of one recently.

I was recently invited on a new podcast to discuss Fitter Confident You from a business perspective plus my backstory, to allow for a deeper dive than is often heard in these chats.

I was honoured to be asked to be part of it - and was in some stellar company among the other guests - and was prepared that it would be more than just a back-patting love-in.

The hosts were great and from the off we got into interesting discussions about why I do what I do, why it's needed and the challenges facing my community.

As you may have gathered by now, I adore what I do; I'm so proud of Fitter Confident You and everyone in it, and I work hard, every single day, to support us all on this journey.

As you will probably also know, I get pretty animated and light up when discussing this, and illustrating why Fitter Confident You is so wonderful and so needed, and how we all help each other progress, build confidence and find our own ways.

Which led to the male host looking a bit put out...

"Well," he said, "now I'm sad... You say you help Gay, Bi, Trans guys who don't feel confident with their fitness or in a gym... but what about me? It makes me sad I'm not included in what you're doing to help people..."

This instantly brought me to a huge fork in the road.

The host is a great coach who I respect and who has helped thousands of people... But knowing he's straight, his moment making it all about him and straight men's problems, is one of the reasons we're all still stuck.

This is how I wish I'd responded...

"I understand why you're feeling like that. The ethos and approach behind Fitter Confident You, of course, can work for anyone. The problem is that the straight man has been in charge in society for hundreds - thousands! - of years. No one is belittling your personal journey and struggles, no one is saying it can't be tough for you to get started with some work-outs, to build confidence in the gym too...

But myself and my community have that AND years of oppression, of living as second-class citizens, of our lives being illegal (until 1967 in the UK).

What would help all of us is for you to pause for a second before saying 'what about me?' because everything has been about you, since the world began.

For you to acknowledge that you may have your individual struggles, but you don't face being shouted at, abused, attacked, just for holding hands with your partner, in the street.

That nowhere in the world is it illegal to be straight, but in 70 countries it's illegal to be gay.

And somewhat mind-bogglingly, in 10 countries, it's punish-able by death.

What you're experiencing now - possibly for the very first time - is exclusion from something that sounds appealing to you.

Imagine a lifetime of being on the outside.

Of being denied basic human and civil rights for hundreds of years - marriage for example.

So yes, you could say that Fitter Confident You does positively discriminate - affirmative action if you want - to reach out to my community and say I've built a safe space where you can be you on your terms. Where you can start to understand how fitness and wellbeing works for you, when there isn't the extra layer of stress, complexity and generational trauma.

But when we've missed out on our own safe spaces, support, even community, is it really a bad thing that these are now being offered?

Yes, I want you to be healthy, happy, strong, fit and confident, I want that for all of us, but you're going to have to find a coach and programme designed for you, because it's not my responsibility to solve your straight man problems."

Of course, it's easy to say this in a book... Only it isn't. Confronting my own fallibility and lack of courage in this instance is uncomfortable, because what I actually said was:

"Oh, but I do work with straight men!"

Which I do and am happy to, but it's not the core drive of FCY.

I acquiesced to make the straight man happy. To avoid any further confrontation or possible challenges to what I do. Which is the same when we're faced with a choice to out ourselves or just float under the radar, and as mentioned, sometimes we just don't have the mental bandwidth to have that conversation again.

So please don't see this as pressure to come out or to be some kind of LGBTQ+ saviour.

When you have the capacity to stand up proudly and boldly, then every word you utter, every eye with which you make and hold contact, is a step forward for us all, into the light.

But when you don't, it's 100% ok to just do what's right for you in that situation. You have to protect your heart and energy first, and after that you can be publicly bold.

How does this relate to fitness?

In spite of me avoiding the confrontation in the interview, over the last 10 years I have found my voice and the courage of my convictions to speak up more than ever before. This is clearly still a work-in-progress, but being a voice for those who can't yet speak is another way to support each other.

This has correlated with me falling head-over-heels in love with fitness, exercise, workouts, but most importantly, what I get out of them. Yes, I love the doing - and if there's no doing, there's no outcome - but I also love all the ways they've helped me grow as a person and get more from every single day.

For example:

▶ Lifting weights forces my body to grow stronger...

▶ Becoming physically stronger allows me to literally do more...

▶ Doing more gives me more life experience, more opportunities to meet and learn from amazing people...

▶ Being around those amazing people brings new perspectives, new ways to look at the world and to understand my place in it...

▶ The more I understand my place in the world, the more I grasp my inherent power, live the life I choose, stand up for those people who need it more than ever and just do more of what I love, for the world around me.

All from picking up some weights and putting them down again - remarkable!

This has also given me the chance to take more personal responsibility for my situation. The more I have done this, the more I've acknowledged my responsibility for my mistakes, habits, times things have gone wrong, *just* as much as any wins, the happier I've been.

This is what I mean by becoming your own cheerleader and own inspiration. What you're doing IS remarkable, and the sooner you become aware of this, the sooner you get to do more remarkable things, and more and more by design too.

To summarise: please always start by pleasing and protecting yourself - that isn't selfish, it's crucial.

Sound the Personal Development Cliché Klaxon, but I can't help but reference how, if a plane loses pressure, we must put on our own oxygen mask first - you can't help anyone if you've passed out, and trust me, you're not very useful if you have passed out.

Not that you have to be useful specifically, but I want you healthy, happy, refreshed, confident, stronger, feeling sexy, and that starts at home, with you understanding it and believing it that little bit more, day by day by day.

Regular workouts and decisions to do good, life-enhancing things for yourself further this, boosting your own world, allowing you to do more of what makes you, you.

If that involves standing a little bit taller, voicing when things could be done differently, then amazing. But that isn't a requirement, I promise. You'll already have an inkling as to what works for you. Trust that intuition, *lean into it,* find your tribe of cheerleaders and life will flow that bit easier each day.

EPILOGUE
TIME TO CATCH UP WITH GEORGE, ONE LAST TIME

SIX MONTHS ON FROM OUR LAST CHECK-IN, LOTS *hasn't* changed for George... But that's the point, things don't need to change as drastically as people often think for there to be big shifts in your life.

He's still at the same company, still with his partner, but they're a bit closer now. This is intangible in some ways, but at the same time, George now has a bit more energy and generally feels a bit brighter. He's more present and active in their relationship. Their sex life has become more exciting and enjoyable and they feel that bit more intimate with each other.

He now exercises two or three times a week. Sometimes it's only once (or not at all!), the big difference is George now doesn't feel bad or guilty when he can't workout - if anything, he misses it (that was a shock!).

This started with home workouts after he bought a pair of 5kg weights from Decathlon - funny how they felt SO heavy that first day, carrying them back to the car from the shop, and now he's lifting three times that, with ease. He found a free workout online to follow along, which he did for the first month, but grew out of it and started thinking something built for him would better support him.

He found an online fitness group for LGBTQ+ people - Fitter Confident Us - which, for the first time, showed him that fitness in the gay community wasn't just about six packs and getting your bodyfat as low as possible. He made connections and while he didn't post anything in the group for the first few months, just being around other guys like him, realising he wasn't alone, was empowering, supportive, and so encouraging.

He started joining in with the group's included Zoom work-out, which also connected him to more people, showing him all different body types, people at all different stages of their fitness journeys and different ways to workout. All which added fuel to his motivation.

After umming and ahhing for a few months, George reached out to the Personal Trainer behind the group to ask about getting a personalised plan. The PT turned out to be friendly and approachable and not the scary, intimidating person he thought all PTs secretly were. They had a chat and after signing up, George received his actually-very-doable plan, which felt like a nice evolution of what he'd started.

The home workouts were a great experience at building his confidence, fitness, and strength at home, away from the looks and stares he believed he'd receive in public... But now, it was time to face that public!

He rejoined the gym he'd signed up for at the start of the year and discovered it also wasn't as scary or intimidating as he'd believed, especially after he'd had his induction and then treated himself to another one-off PT session, so he could double check he was happy with the various bits of equipment.

After a month he tried a class. The first one was a bit nerve-wracking (as he was late and had to go right at the front, in full view of both the trainer and the class), but he quite enjoyed the positive energy and group motivation. What's been interesting is noticing the more things he tries (fitness-wise and in other parts of his life) the easier it is to keep trying other things.

He kept his home workout weights because they're handy if he doesn't have the time to go to the gym - also, sentimental attachment to the kit that helped him exercise consistently.

Speaking of which, it felt very strange to not be spending hours on cardio machines - could 20 minutes lifting weights and using resistance machines really be doing the same (or even a better) job?

Turns out, it can! But more than that, because the workouts are shorter, more efficient and because he's enjoying how they make him feel (buzzing, some days, as opposed to mentally and physically destroyed after an hour on the treadmill and bike) - it all makes staying the course much easier too.

Like Alessandro mentioned, he now understands a bit more about food and how it works for him. Pushing aside the guilt around a big meal or weekends out can still sometimes feel tough, but he's working on that too.

He learned how to track his calories at the start, which was also something he'd heard about and avoided, thinking it would take the fun out of food or take over his life. Neither was true, it simply helped him see that some foods are a lot more calorie-dense than others. He drank a bit more water which he found surprisingly filling, and even tried a protein shake... Which wasn't for him! But he tried it and was proud of himself for that.

He still eats pizza and drinks wine and sometimes comfort-eats chocolate when particularly stressed, but he's much more aware of this now, and again, is much kinder to himself when it happens, which is going a long way to break the cycle of guilt > stress > eat > guilt > stress > eat...

George is sleeping a bit better too, which has meant he's had more energy, a more stable mood and a bit less anxiety. Steadily, this has begun to help George see himself differently. He has greater self-belief - partly from realising and noticing the physical progress he's made with his workouts - another intangible, but there's something inspiring about lifting heavier weights - a certain self-reliance has grown. Partly from just not feeling as sluggish physically or brain-fogged mentally - his body moves a bit more freely and he's that bit happier with who he sees in the mirror.

What's really surprised him is how his growing confidence and energy has trickled over into his working life.

George speaks up that bit more and is much more protective of his time and boundaries - not allowing meetings to be booked over lunchtime (when he now goes to the gym) or at the end of the day (so he can leave at a reasonable time and switch off).

His clothes fit differently too. He's gone down a belt loop and losing a bit of weight around his middle has helped his posture too. Of course, he sometimes still has long days at the office when his shoulders round and he slumps in his seat, but now he's aware of it and sits up straighter and goes for a walk when possible.

There have been a few naysayers along the way, some easier to deal with than others, starting with office life - there were some looks when he politely refused the cake that had been brought in, and even some jibes from friends when he chose a different drink when they met up one night.

Harder to manage was his Mum.

"You look fine!"

"I read that exercise is actually worse for you overall."

"Will I have to cook health food for you now?!"

And it was difficult not to hurt her feelings at first. Looking back, he can see that on one level she equated her love with the food she made and served, so by rejecting her food, he was rejecting her; George just had to steadily reassure her that there was no ulterior motive to eating a regular size serving of her food and turning down seconds.

He knows what she says isn't mean - she was suckered into the Diet Industry at its most bizarre, the 70s and 80s, and was always on a diet.

There was the Cabbage Soup Diet:

"Eat only cabbage soup for three weeks and you'll lose weight!"

No shit! You'll also die from malnutrition and starvation.

There was the Grapefruit Diet:

"You can eat whatever you want as long as you eat half a grapefruit beforehand!"

But of course! Grapefruit is kryptonite to calories and literally just destroys them!!!

George remembers at one point in his childhood, she stuck a picture on the family fridge of two people on a beach wearing bikinis who she saw as the enemy (in her mind, carrying more weight than they should be). This picture was only stuck there to stop HER from opening the fridge to snack, but it definitely stuck with young George and informed his early beliefs about thin being good and fat being bad.

She's still sceptical, but mentions it less now.

George's partner was also dubious about what he started.

Outwardly, he said he didn't want to eat different foods at different times or be guilted into exercising - which of course, George never did.

Inwardly, he worried that George was getting bored with him or worse, seeing someone else.

The funny thing was, after a few months of the small changes George was making, he started going for walks... Which became jog-walks, which became jogs, which became runs, which became trying the local Park Run, which became joining a local running group.

Maybe a rising tide *does* lift all boats?!

George is now fitter and people have commented on his confidence too, though he still has wobbles sometimes, but he's definitely not where he was at the start of the year.

Another surprise is that the numbers of the scales haven't changed that much - a few kilos down, but nothing at first glance to write home about... But his body shape HAS changed; his waist is a bit trimmer, and he just noticed that his favourite shirt is a bit tight across his shoulders.

He also feels lighter and has less back ache, and now makes time for his fitness and wellbeing.

So while not much has changed... Actually, everything has, but in such a kind, slow, steady and sustainable way that it never felt too much and it just supported George in feeling better, day by day.

A Fitter Confident George, or even a Fitter Confident YOU.

UNBORING GLOSSARY OF TERMS

Bleep Test

School-sanctioned method to torture PE classes, ostensibly to determine the pupil's fitness level, but with little real use apart from bragging rights of the top performing children.

Body Mass Index (BMI)

Method of determining someone's 'health' and if they're carrying more fat than they 'should' based on very specific parameters - most commonly used by the medical profession.

I'm not a fan of BMI as it fails to take into account muscle mass, bone density, overall body composition and racial and sex differences, yet it spits out a number and a colour-coding, making people panic.

Also, there are no grey areas either. You're in one category, lose 1kg and now you're in a different category, so it doesn't encourage long term, sustainable change, instead it just pushes people to diet and exercise as quickly as possible to bring the numbers down enough to get into a healthier group. Very unFCY! So people may get out of the 'obese' category, but only just, and still think that's enough, purely because they've gone down a band.

Cardiovascular Training (Cardio / CV)

Any exercise that increases the heart rate and breathing to increase blood flow and oxygen through the body. Running! Dance classes! Swimming! Cycling! Brisk walking! Scrolling through Twitter!

All lovely and all health- and fitness-improving. Plus, there is something about a cardio workout that can really help to clear the mind and clear out negative thoughts.

The issue is for years, we've been led to believe that cardio is the only real approach should you want to burn fat, when it's really quite low down the list for that - all exercise is.

The number one way to elicit small and sustainable fat loss is by consistently eating a bit less, creating a calorie deficit, where you're eating slightly less than you need. Much easier to stick to than starving yourself and much easy to achieve than through fitness - especially cardio - alone.

Cheat Day / Cheat Meal

A carrot dangled as an incentive for 'eating well' all week, or 'sticking to a diet'. I.e., if you're 'good' you can then be 'bad' and eat what you want. The problem is, this compartmentalises your food as 'good' or 'bad', 'fun' or 'tedious'. Of course, if you only see food as a chore, or plain, or restrictive, then an incentive might be the only way to stick to your plan - but this isn't sustainable, and you are not a spaniel who needs training!

If you want a 'treat' / food you enjoy, please just have it - making your food intake contingent on your behaviour can lead to disordered eating and adds stress to your meals, when it really doesn't have to be that way.

Compound Exercises (see also Isolation Exercises)

Any exercise that uses more than one muscle group and joint. For example, squats, which require your legs, bum and core at a minimum (and whole upper body too if you hold a weight or have a bar on your back!).

Compound exercises are more tiring as they use more of you all at once, but that also means they're more efficient and stimulate more muscle fibres for every rep. The main compound exercises are:

- Squats (legs, bum, core, upper body)
- Lunges (legs, bum, core, upper body)
- Deadlifts - picking a weight off the ground and putting it down (legs, bum, core, upper body)
- Bench/Chest press (Chest, arms, core)
- Strict/Shoulder press (shoulders, arms, core)

Learning these five moves will stand you in good stead for any workout in the future, and you'll always be able to have a good workout with these moves alone.

Diets

Diets don't work. Not long term. The 'Diet and Weight Management' Industry in the United States is worth more than $72.6 BILLION a year (Globe NewsWire https://bit.-ly/3NWVyhw). Which is great and really paying off because the United States is one of the healthiest and fittest nations on earth!!!

Clearly, there's a global problem going on here, I only singled out the US as their stats were easy to find.

Here's why diets don't work and why people yo-yo diet so frequently: Diets only teach you how to eat and live... on the diet, i.e., according to the diet's strict rules and restrictions. When you stop adhering to its rules, you haven't learned how to eat and live in the real world, and most people revert to their old habits and patterns of eating.

The Fitter Confident You approach is the opposite of a diet. I'll never ask you to give up any of your favourite foods or starve yourself, because you don't need to.

It works because you learn how it all works, with no guilt or pressure, and it allows you to start making informed choices that support your goals. At the start, you don't even really need to change what you eat, just make small liveable modifications to how you eat.

DOMS

This is the ache you get 24-72hrs after a workout and stands for Delayed Onset Muscle Soreness. I know, the first time it happens it's a bit of a shock, but it's very rarely that bad again and ultimately, it's a good thing. It means your body has done something it hasn't done before (or for a while), which means it has to adapt to it. And it adapts to it by getting stronger and better able to cope with it next time.

Of course, what your body *doesn't* know, is that over time, you're going to increase the weights again, try different exercises, different workouts, and yes, the DOMS will show up again... But you never forget your first DOMS...!

Dumbbells and Barbells

The main equipment in the 'Free Weights' area of your gym. Dumbbells are the ones you hold in one hand each. You will usually find a rack of various fixed weight dumbbells and in most gyms I've been to, these will never, ever be in the right order!

Barbells are the long bars (usually either 15kg or 20kg - check on the end of each one where it usually tells you which) to which you can add additional weights, in the form of plates - literally plate-shaped weights of varying increments.

Fitter Confident Younicorn

You! Yep, that's right. Just by reading this book, you are now, officially, a Fitter Confident Younicorn - I don't make the rules up! (Actually, round these parts, I do, but they're good rules, I promise.)

A Fitter Confident Younicorn knows that there are no quick fixes, no shortcuts to their fitness, strength, health, happiness and confidence progressing... BUT they also know it never has to be a slog or a chore. They do good things for themselves and when they can't - i.e., when work gets particularly busy - they just get back to doing the good things, with no guilt that they are behind or need to catch up.

They also cheer everyone else on and take joy in the act of doing so. They encourage the beginners who are just dipping their toes and the ones who have been doing this for much longer, and do so for the love of supporting their fellow Younicorns.

Once you become one, you'll be amazed how much easier everything associated with your fitness and wellbeing becomes. You'll also start bumping into them, all over the place - this is a movement with heart and the kindest, most inclusive community you'll find.

Fitter Confident Youniverse

Here! You're already here!

The creation of the Fitter Confident Youniverse was easy: whatever the traditional Fitness Industry did, or has always done, I'd do the opposite.

Moody and serious, black and white photos of both PTs and clients in pain and fighting with their workouts? No thanks!

An exclusive boys club, designed to be intimidating and keep most people out? Definitely not!

Promotional campaigns shaming people for their body and focusing on appearance only? Not in the Fitter Confident Youniverse!

As I had felt excluded from fitness and gyms growing up, I knew the Fitter Confident Youniverse had to be as inclusive, welcoming, kind and encouraging as possible, if it was going to make a difference and actually start to change things. While the Fitter Confident Youniverse has specifically been created to support the LGBTQ+ in fitness, the principles and methods apply to everyone, and I firmly believe that one of the ways we improve life on earth for all of us is through fitness, wellbeing and taking a smidge of personal responsibility in creating our own health futures.

Futureproofing

A client said this to me as their way of describing what they were doing by working with me, and I LOVED it. It gives a much greater purpose and drive to what we do, and means clients have a combination of short and long term goals. While the future can sometimes feel like a distant land we'll never reach, if we pause and look around us, we'll see people who didn't understand the gift of a bit of fitness, a bit of wellbeing, and in their 60s, 70s, and later, aren't able to do what they want to do, as their bodies don't work how they'd wish.

While exercising and a bit of nutrition knowledge aren't a magic elixir of life, they will contribute to you being stronger, more confident, healthier, getting ill less frequently and just being able to keep living your life how you want to live it.

Good / Bad food

There's no such thing. Food is neither good or bad. Some have greater (or fewer!) amounts of nutrients and are more (or less!) calorie-dense, but it's us, as humans, that infer that any food is 'good' or 'bad', based on all the things we've learned and experienced through life, which is just silly. It's just food.

Additionally, you haven't been 'bad' when you've eaten certain foods... But neither have you been good when you've had a salad for lunch either!

Gymfidence

The confidence that comes from working out - it absolutely does not require a gym membership, it just makes the word sound good. Gymfidence grows quicker than most people expect, from two things:

1. Underestimating how quickly exercise can make you feel good (it really can!)
2. Overestimating how scary people in gyms actually are (they're really not, but I know this is a journey that takes all of us different lengths of time).

High Intensity Interval Training (HIIT)

Jumping around lots in the name of fitness... I jest. The principles of HIIT are sound and will contribute to your overall fitness and yes, burn some fat and strengthen your muscles. The biggest part of fitness is finding what you enjoy, and if it's HIIT classes and workouts, that's awesome; that means you'll make time for them and stick to them and progress.

The downside for me is they can seem too intense to an outsider, so may not always be as welcoming as they could be. Plus, it's only a very small percentage of the population who enjoy burpees, so as a method to encourage people into a fitness class, it seems a bit backwards!

Isolation Exercises (see also Compound Exercises)

These literally 'isolate' one muscle while working out.

A classic example is the bicep curl, which works... your bicep! Excellent deduction! These smaller moves are generally classes as accessory work, and should really be bolted on to the compound moves.

Macronutrients - Carbohydrate, Fat, Protein (and alcohol!)

These are the three (or four!) essential nutrient components in all our food. I put alcohol in brackets as technically it *is* a macronutrient, but (and apologies for the Personal Trainer cliché coming up) it's empty calories - there is no benefit to consumption of alcohol (well, apart from delicious taste and fun, but you know what I mean).

136

That doesn't mean you need to cut it out, but forewarned is forearmed. If a client has been sticking to their sensible Fitter Confident You nutrition coaching but knocking back bottles of red wine at the weekend and not including their calories, then it can be easy to spot what needs adjusting for them to make the progress they're after.

You may have heard of 'macros' or people 'tracking their macros', and while this can be a useful tool in our toolbox, it's unnecessary for most people and certainly not needed at the start of your Fitter Confident You journey. An understanding of the right amount of food (calories) for you to eat and a slightly higher protein intake is pretty much all it takes to help you burn some fat, support some muscle growth and feel less bloated.

No food need ever be off-limits - food is a joy and I want you to go on enjoying all the different types we have available to us. Cutting out an entire food group - the classic one is carbs - isn't healthy, isn't tasty and will just give you a withdrawal headache and hate the process. Small reductions in the amounts you're eating is far more sustainable, far kinder and far easier to start and stick to.

Resistance Training

NOW we're talking. If I had to choose one fitness approach for life - and that's what I'm essentially going to do now - I would go for resistance training aka, weight lifting in some form.

I know that phrase puts some people off, so allow me to elaborate: weight training doesn't just mean using weights, because YOU can be the weight too! Bodyweight workouts, using resistance bands and suspension straps (known sometimes by the brand name TRX) and any other kit you find at home or in a gym that forces your body to work against - you got it - resistance!

It has almost infinite benefits but to list a few:

- Stimulate and build muscle - creating a strong body that lets you do what you want to do. PLUS, muscle takes more energy/calories to support than any other tissue in your body, so you'll burn more calories just at rest and it gets easier to stay lean (if that's your goal)
- Reduced incidences of chronic illnesses - cancer, heart disease, diabetes, osteoporosis
- Improves balance and coordination (so you'll be less likely to fall over)
- Improves bone density (should you fall over, you'll be less likely to break a bone)
- Improves and supports posture and can help reduce back aches and pains
- Of all the workouts, weight-lifting causes you to burn the most amount of energy/calories *after* a workout too
- Personally, there's nothing quite like hitting a personal best achievement in your favourite move - maybe a squat or a chest press (I have also experienced running-based achievements and they're

great too, but feeling stronger and more physically capable is the one for me).

Rest / Rest Days

When it's all firing and you're working out regularly and things are coming together, the logical way to progress things is to just do it all more... But very little with fitness and health progress is linear or 100% logical.

You might be in a groove with your health and fitness, working out four times a week, seeing and feeling progress and changes and feeling better each week. It's admirable that you want to keep pushing, but remember that bodies need rest to recover and specifically, grow.

While a workout might give you a muscle pump, that's just extra blood in the muscles making them swell. They haven't grown there and then, that comes when you rest and feed yourself appropriately. Before you add another workout day, I'd ensure you had been increasing the weights you're lifting. This is a much easier way to encourage progress - or bust through a plateau. The rule of thumb is to increase the weights you lift in each session - even by just 1lb / 500g - but anything more than your body has had to face... is more than your body has had to face! So, it has to respond by growing back bigger, fitter, stronger.

So, nudge your weights up next workout before you add an extra workout day, as your rest days are so important for physical and mental recovery.

Sets and Repetitions (reps)

The number of times you're aiming to perform a certain exercise. For example, if your plan says '3 x 10 bodyweight squats', this means three sets of 10 repetitions of a squat, done without any additional weights.

You would do 10 repetitions of the squat - 10 squats in a row, then rest, that's set one.

You would then do a second set of 10 squats in a row, then rest.

And then a final set of 10 squats - and that's your three sets of 10 reps - great start!

Six Pack

Mythical source of all male happiness.

Here's the thing, you have one! If you didn't, you wouldn't be able to sit or stand upright (it's also known as your rectus abdominis muscle). All six packs are various states of conditioning (how strong they are) and how clearly they've been revealed - which, yes, is down to reducing belly fat.

I can guarantee you that 'having one' (by which, I mean having a low enough body fat percentage for it to show) will not make you any happier than you are now, if you focus just on the desire to have one. If you're able to celebrate the processes, the things you learned, the journey, the ups and down, your overall evolution and view the revealing of your six pack as one of the many, MANY amazing things that happen when we turn our focus on ourselves, then yes, you will be a happier, fitter, confident individual. But a six pack is far from the be all and end all of happiness.

Supersets (and Giant Sets!)

As a way to make workouts tougher (and sometimes just to make them more interesting!) exercises can be combined together. For example, if your plan says '3 x 10 bodyweight squats, 3 x 10 push-ups', you would do:

10 repetitions of the squat, and then with as little rest as possible, 10 push-ups, then you get to rest.

Then you'd do another 10 squats and another 10 push-ups, then rest.

And finally, another 10 squats and another 10 push-ups, then you're done - great work!

A Giant Set is simply three (or more!) exercises stacked together, performed one after the other before you rest.

Weight Loss

What people say when they really mean 'fat loss'. I understand why people might avoid using the word fat, but if we're being precise, weight loss implies that your goal is to lose any weight - doesn't matter what - as long as the number on the scales reduces.

The problem is that we don't want to lose any weight, and when people starve themselves for this goal, yes, there will be fat loss, but there will also be muscle loss, which isn't a healthy goal. Neither will it support a long term strong healthy body. Weight loss at any cost is a really unhealthy approach and not something taught or encouraged in the Fitter Confident Youniverse.

We avoid this by only reducing our food intake a little - the upshot is this makes sticking to it, and therefore achieving consistency, much easier. We also encourage weight-lifting to stimulate your muscles and preserve muscle as much as possible. On top of this, a higher protein intake (than most people generally have) also contributes to muscle maintenance, keeping you lean and strong.

THANKS

Matt Boyles created Fitter Confident You... and I'm so happy I did!

Realising the benefits that I'd enjoyed firsthand, and also realising that there were most likely other people in my community who felt like I used to was the starting point. But the way the Fitter Confident Youniverse has grown and evolved, and all the wonderful people I've come into contact with, has made the last five years my most enjoyable, productive and successful (in a million different ways).

So firstly, thank you to every single Fitter Confident Younicorn. You inspire and encourage me every day, and I couldn't do it without you.

Thank you to my amazing family for your unerring support and love. It means the world and I'm so grateful for you all.

Thank you to my partner Tom and all my friends for the love and belief... But also for putting up with me bang on about fitness, and younicorns and live workouts and capybaras and all the other things I've been known to get excited about.

Big thanks also to Lisa Johnson, my amazing mentor, for the opportunity and encouragement to write this book.

And thank you to Abigail Horne, Lucy Crane, Deanne Adams, Celestin Dimitriu and all at Authors & Co for your wisdom, guidance and kicks up the bum as needed to get it done!

ABOUT THE AUTHOR

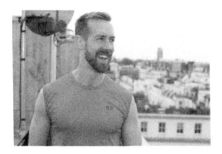

Matt Boyles is the Founder and CEO of Fitter Confident You. 15 years ago, he would have laughed at the idea that he would be running a successful online fitness business but that right there is the gift of fitness.

Discovering the power of fitness, looking after yourself a bit more and all the associated good habits that it instills, changed his life, health, mindset and career-trajectory... And this is how Fitter Confident You helps its community, by supporting anyone who wants to build their strength and find their voice and confidence.

Fitter Confident You has helped more than 1,400 LGBTQ+ clients around the world build strength of mind, body and overall resilience... And we're not stopping there!

Head over to www.fitterconfidentyou.net/12weekFCY to start your Fitter Confident journey today.

FB group:

https://www.facebook.com/groups/1857669824451809

facebook.com/fitteryouglobal

twitter.com/fitteryouglobal

instagram.com/fitteryouglobal

youtube.com/FitterConfidentYou

linkedin.com/in/matt-boyles-he-him-3aa6415

LET'S KEEP IN TOUCH!

There are so many ways Fitter Confident You can support you, at whatever stage of your fitness journey you find yourself.

Fitter Confident Us is my amazing membership, to inspire action, motivation and progress in a kind, supportive environment. It includes weekly workouts, regular yoga sessions, mindset training, the FCY Book Club and getting to hang out with the most supportive community there is - www.fittercon fidentyou.net/fitterconfidentus

Ready to step it up? Good for you! The 12-week flagship Fitter Confident You plan is fully personalised for your success, built around what you need to finally stick to and enjoy a workout plan AND includes all the Fitter Confident Us goodies above, too! www.fitterconfidentyou.net/12weekfcy

You'll find me as @fitteryouglobal on all the social platforms you fancy! Follow along for fitness with humour, heart and personality.

Finally, the Albert Kennedy Trust, who I mentioned right at the start, is here: www.akt.org.uk/. The Trust focuses on LGBTQ+ youth homelessness, which has risen dramatically in the last few years, helping young people into training, education, employment and safe housing. I'm so proud to be a supporter and as a reminder, £1 from the sale of each copy of this book goes straight to them, so thank you!

Printed in Great Britain
by Amazon

84823324R00089